Full-Body Flexibility

SECOND EDITION

Jay Blahnik

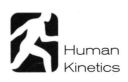
Human
Kinetics

Library of Congress Cataloging-in-Publication Data

Blahnik, Jay.
  Full-body flexibility / Jay Blahnik. -- 2nd ed.
    p. cm.
  ISBN-13: 978-0-7360-9036-0 (soft cover)
  ISBN-10: 0-7360-9036-3 (soft cover)
  1. Stretching exercises. I. Title.
  RA781.63.B56 2010
  613.7'1--dc22

                        2010023384

ISBN-10: 0-7360-9036-3 (print)
ISBN-13: 978-0-7360-9036-0 (print)

This publication is written and published to provide accurate and authoritative information relevant to the subject matter presented. It is published and sold with the understanding that the author and publisher are not engaged in rendering legal, medical, or other professional services by reason of their authorship or publication of this work. If medical or other expert assistance is required, the services of a competent professional person should be sought.

Acquisitions Editor: Justin Klug; **Developmental Editor:** Carla Zych; **Assistant Editors:** Michael Bishop and Elizabeth Evans; **Copyeditor:** John Wentworth; **Graphic Designer:** Nancy Rasmus; **Graphic Artist:** Julie L. Denzer; **Cover Designer:** Keith Blomberg; **Photographer (cover and interior):** Stephen Ryan Photographies; **Photo Asset Manager:** Laura Fitch; **Visual Production Assistant:** Joyce Brumfield; **Photo Production Manager:** Jason Allen; **Art Manager:** Kelly Hendren; **Associate Art Manager:** Alan L. Wilborn; **Illustrator:** © Human Kinetics; **Printer:** United Graphics

We thank Stephen Ryan of Stephen Ryan Photographies in Lake Forest, CA, for assistance in providing the location for the photo shoot for this book.

Human Kinetics books are available at special discounts for bulk purchase. Special editions or book excerpts can also be created to specification. For details, contact the Special Sales Manager at Human Kinetics.

Printed in the United States of America   10 9 8 7 6 5 4 3 2

The paper in this book is certified under a sustainable forestry program.

Human Kinetics
Web site: www.HumanKinetics.com

United States: Human Kinetics
P.O. Box 5076
Champaign, IL 61825-5076
800-747-4457
e-mail: humank@hkusa.com

Canada: Human Kinetics
475 Devonshire Road Unit 100
Windsor, ON N8Y 2L5
800-465-7301 (in Canada only)
e-mail: info@hkcanada.com

Europe: Human Kinetics
107 Bradford Road
Stanningley
Leeds LS28 6AT, United Kingdom
+44 (0) 113 255 5665
e-mail: hk@hkeurope.com

Australia: Human Kinetics
57A Price Avenue
Lower Mitcham, South Australia 5062
08 8372 0999
e-mail: info@hkaustralia.com

New Zealand: Human Kinetics
P.O. Box 80
Torrens Park, South Australia 5062
0800 222 062
e-mail: info@hknewzealand.com

E5064

This book is dedicated to my parents, David and Charlene Blahnik.
I love you with all my heart.

contents

part I   Total-Body Stretch System

part II   Regions of Flexibility

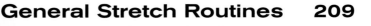

part III   **Fitness and Sport Routines**

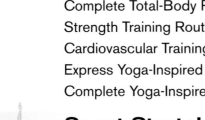 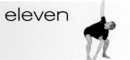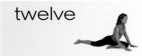

stretch finder

> *continued*

stretch finder > *continued*

> continued

stretch finder > *continued*

	Active or Passive	Neck	Shoulders	Arms	Hands	Chest	Back	Abdominals	Quadriceps	Hamstrings	Glutes & Hips	Inner Thighs	Calves	Shins	Feet	Page number
Chapter 6																
Lying Leg Raise	P									X						118
One-Leg Hip Hinge	P									X						119
Double-Leg Hip Hinge	P									X						120
Standing Leg Raise	P									X						121
Dynamic Knee Kick	A									X						122
Dynamic Lying Leg Raise	A									X						123
Dynamic Lying Knee Kick	A									X						124
Dynamic Seated Knee Kick	A									X						125
Dynamic Rolling Ball Knee Kick	A									X						126
Dynamic Rolling Ball Hip Hinge	P									X						127
Hip Hinge (Ball)	P									X						128
Chapter 7																
Heel Drop	P												X			130
Heel Press	P												X			131
Toe Up	P												X			132
Seated Stretch-Strap Foot Pull	P												X			133
Dynamic Seated Flex and Point	A												X			134
Dynamic Heel Drop	P												X			135
Seated Thinker Pose	P												X			136
Bent-Knee Heel Drop	P												X			137
Bent-Knee Heel Press	P												X			138
Dynamic Bent-Knee Heel Press	P												X			139

REGIONS AFFECTED

	Active or Passive	Neck	Shoulders	Arms	Hands	Chest	Back	Abdominals	Quadriceps	Hamstrings	Glutes & Hips	Inner Thighs	Calves	Shins	Feet	Page number
						REGIONS AFFECTED										
Dynamic Seated Bent-Knee Flex and Point	A												X			140
Toe Drop	P													X		141
Seated Foot Pull	P													X		142
Kneeling Toe Point and Sit	P													X		143
Dynamic Seated Half-Circle	A													X		144
Dynamic Seated Ankle Pull	P													X		145
Dynamic Seated Ankle Roll	A													X		146
Seated Foot Massage	P														X	147
Dynamic Seated Toe Flex and Point	A														X	148
Dynamic Seated Toe Wiggle	A														X	149
Chapter 8																
Lying Spinal Twist	P					X	X				X					152
Triangle	P						X					X				153
Extended Angle	P						X					X				154
Warrior	P							X			X					155
Chair	A							X			X		X		X	156
Downward-Facing Dog	P					X		X	X				X			157
Upward-Facing Dog	P							X			X			X		158
Child's Pose	P		X				X		X							159
Forward Bend	P						X			X						160
Fan	P						X			X		X				161
Sitting Angular Leg Extension	P						X			X		X				162

> continued

stretch finder > continued

	Active or Passive	Neck	Shoulders	Arms	Hands	Chest	Back	Abdominals	Quadriceps	Hamstrings	Glutes & Hips	Inner Thighs	Calves	Shins	Feet	Page number
															REGIONS AFFECTED	
Dynamic Leg Kick	A						X			X	X					188
Dynamic Cross-Knee Squat	A						X			X	X	X				189
Dynamic Squat Twist Reach	A		X			X	X			X	X					190
Dynamic Cross-Reach	A						X					X				191
Dynamic Lunge and Push Back	P										X					192
Dynamic Single-Side Bow	A		X			X		X	X		X					193
Dynamic Lunge and Twist	A						X	X				X				194
Dynamic Squat Reach Twist	A					X	X	X		X	X					195
Dynamic Knee Circle Twist	A						X	X			X	X				196
Dynamic Child's Pose and Camel	A		X			X		X	X		X					197
Dynamic Hip Swivel and Chest Lift	A							X			X	X				198
Dynamic Roll and Reach	A						X			X	X					199
Dynamic Squat Twist and Hinge	A						X	X		X	X					200
Dynamic Knee Lift and Leg Back	A									X	X					201
Dynamic Lateral Reach Slide	A						X	X				X				202
Dynamic Figure 8	A										X	X				203
Dynamic Knee Bend and Hug	A								X	X	X					204
Dynamic Lunge and Circle	A						X	X				X				205

preface

Stretching has come a long way since the first edition of *Full-Body Flexibility*. We always knew how important it was to stretch, but most of us didn't do it as much as we should. And when we did do it we didn't always do it in the most effective manner, often relying on a few old-fashioned stretches we learned when we were kids from our teachers or coaches.

In fact, one of the reasons I wrote the first edition of this book was to provide a simple resource that might nudge people to stretch more often and to do it a bit smarter. My goal was to highlight a common-sense approach to stretching that was easy to understand but that was also based on the most current research and expert opinions.

Although we are probably still not stretching as often as we should, the rise in popularity of activities such as yoga has brought stretching to the forefront of the fitness movement. In addition, coaches, personal trainers, and exercise experts have begun to intensify their efforts to get their athletes, clients, and students to make stretching a bigger part of their overall training routines, which often results in marked improvements in performance and injury prevention. Even better, there is growing agreement about the best time, the best methods, and the best approach to stretching. Stretching is finally on its way to becoming as significant in people's training regimes as the other components of fitness.

With this in mind, I felt it was the perfect time to release the second edition of *Full-Body Flexibility*. I have many new stretches to share, and my stretch system has become more refined since the first edition. In addition, I was able to expand the page count to include more of the multiregion stretches inspired by yoga that have become so popular as well as many more of the multidimensional, dynamic stretches that are ideal for sport conditioning and training. The routines from the first edition that readers loved have been retained in this new edition, but they have been updated, expanded, and refreshed to provide even better results.

The three-step stretch system I present in chapter 2 is worth reading because it provides you with a unique but simple method for stretching that will improve your flexibility, mobility, and strength in ways you can see, feel, and truly benefit from.

Once you have learned the three-step system, you will find 175 individual stretches (almost double the amount in the first edition!) to help you target the areas that need stretching the most. I have divided the body into regions to make it easy to locate a muscle group or stretch and to understand the benefits. I have also included chapters on multiregion (yoga-inspired) stretches and sport mobility stretches that incorporate multiple muscle groups at once and that are generally more advanced than other stretches. With so many individual stretches to choose from, along with my three-step stretch system, you will have more information than you will ever need to stretch your body effectively and in a variety of ways.

If you want more structure, the 23 stretch routines found in part III of the book make it easy for you to stretch anywhere or anytime. The fitness routines are organized in a way that makes it quick and easy for you to get a good stretch workout. The sport routines provide you with the proper performance and recovery stretches for dozens of sports. The specialty routines allow you to focus on one area of the body or stretch with a specific goal in mind. All the routines use the stretches found in part II of the book. Each routine provides a thumbnail photo of each stretch and a page reference in case you need to look up a stretch while doing one of the routines.

I encourage you to use this book in whatever way most easily fits into your life. If you don't have much time during your day, select a stretch per day at random from the book and just do what you can. Some stretches take only seconds but still provide you with great benefit. If you have more time, explore the routines in the back of the book designed to provide more specific results. Whether you are searching to improve your overall fitness or sport performance or just looking for a more effective way to stretch, *Full-Body Flexibility* gives you the right tools to reduce the tension in your muscles, increase your strength, lubricate your joints, refresh your body, make it easier to reach and bend for things, improve your posture, enhance your athleticism, and help you stand taller.

I have always enjoyed stretching, whether I am doing it to release tension, improve my flexibility, recover from a tough training session, or simply to make it easier to get through my day. When I am unable to stretch regularly, I notice it in how I feel, move, and perform. Then when I get back on my regular stretch routine, I'm freshly amazed by what a difference it makes. As I get older, I also notice how truly helpful stretching is for keeping me limber, strong, and energetic.

Full-Body Flexibility is designed to make it comfortable, quick, and easy to include stretching in your training program or sport performance regime and your day-to-day life. This second edition incorporates the best stretches and best routines into a practical system that will change your understanding of what stretching can do for you.

acknowledgments

The writer of any book usually gets most of the credit. However, anyone who has written a book will tell you that it takes a whole group of people to bring a book to life. It is impossible for me to fully express the gratitude I feel toward these people, but my heart is as grateful as it can be.

First, and always first, I thank God for His many blessings.

Thanks also to the following people:

The staff at Human Kinetics, especially Justin Klug and Carla Zych, who provided direction for my ideas, were patient when I missed my deadlines, and did a superb job of editing this book.

Phil Arney, my business partner and friend, who performed every stretch, provided feedback on every routine, and helped me write (and rewrite) many of the instructions. As always, he was encouraging, supportive, and focused on details I would have otherwise missed. This book would never have been completed without his involvement and support.

Julz Arney and Julie LaFond, my business partners and friends, who provided tremendous initial feedback and direction on the first edition of this book and whose amazing contributions remain an important part of this second edition.

Ben Rubin, MD, the most talented doctor, surgeon, and health professional I know, who has assisted me through multiple strains, pains, and injuries through the years and provided me with world-class advice and exercise information that has helped me beyond measure.

Joel Mackes, Fernanda Rocha, Maria Hamilton, and Audri Geary, the models in the photos of this book, who provided their gorgeous faces, bodies, and hearts to this project and made every stretch look simply incredible.

Renee Woolver and Janis McDuffie, whose expert hair and makeup work enhanced the models' natural beauty.

Steve Ryan, the photographer, who once again provided his exceptional talent and eye to ensure that each photo in the book is clear and beautiful.

part I

Total-Body Stretch System

Stretching Basics

Three-Step Stretch System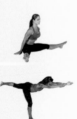

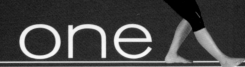

Stretching Basics

If you're like me, you're eager to get going and would rather skip the reading and jump right into a few stretches. But before you dive in, please take the time to read this chapter. It won't take long, and it will provide you with a clear understanding of the approach to stretching outined in this book. Reading this chapter will also help you maximize the benefits of the information, graphics, and photos presented in the book. You will probably need to read this chapter only once, and I assure you it is worth it.

Stretching Techniques and Terms

First let's review a few important techniques and terms. Even if you're familiar with stretching, it's a good idea to double-check your knowledge of this information. Some of these terms are commonly confused and misused.

Static Stretching

Static stretching means a stretch is held in a challenging but comfortable position for a period of time, usually somewhere between 10 to 30 seconds. Static stretching is the most common form of stretching found in general fitness and is considered safe and effective for improving overall flexibility. However, many experts consider static stretching much less beneficial than dynamic stretching for improving range of motion for functional movement, including sports and activities for daily living.

Dynamic Stretching

Dynamic stretching means a stretch is performed by moving through a challenging but comfortable range of motion repeatedly, usually 10 to 12 times. Although dynamic stretching requires more thoughtful coordination than static stretching (because of the movement involved), it is gaining favor among athletes, coaches, trainers, and physical therapists because of its apparent benefits in improving functional range of motion and mobility in sports and activities for daily living.

Note that dynamic stretching should not be confused with old-fashioned ballistic stretching (remember the bouncing toe touches from PE classes?). Dynamic stretching is controlled, smooth, and deliberate, whereas ballistic stretching is uncontrolled, erratic, and jerky. Although there are unique benefits to ballistic stretches, they should be done only under the supervision of a professional because, for most people, the risks of ballistic stretching far outweigh the benefits.

Passive Stretching

Passive stretching means you're using some sort of outside assistance to help you achieve a stretch. This assistance could be your body weight, a strap, leverage, gravity, another person, or a stretching device. With passive stretching, you relax the muscle you're trying to stretch and rely on the external force to hold you in place. You don't usually have to work very hard to do a passive stretch, but there is always the risk that the external force will be stronger than you are flexible, which could cause injury.

Active Stretching

Active stretching means you're stretching a muscle by actively contracting the muscle in opposition to the one you're stretching. You do not use your body weight, a strap, leverage, gravity, another person, or a stretching device. With active stretching, you relax the muscle you're trying to stretch and rely on the opposing muscle to initiate the stretch. Active stretching can be challenging because of the muscular force required to generate the stretch but is generally considered lower risk because you are controlling the stretch force with your own strength rather than an external force.

Every stretch is static or dynamic *and* passive or active, as illustrated in the examples shown in table 1.1.

You might hear or read about other techniques and terms used in stretching (especially by coaches and athletes), such as proprioceptive neuromuscular facilitation (PNF) stretching or active isolated stretching. These techniques are all simply variations of these four types of stretches.

TABLE 1.1 Stretching Technique Classifications

	Static	Dynamic
Passive	Static-passive calf stretch	Dynamic-passive calf stretch
Active	Static-active calf stretch	Dynamic-active stretch

Most of the stretches you see and do are likely static-passive stretches. Static-passive stretches are the most common stretches and the easiest to perform. If executed with good technique, these stretches are effective in improving flexibility and range of motion.

However, most experts now agree that although static-passive stretches have many benefits, it's best to do more dynamic-active stretches. Because dynamic-active stretches require you to use and build your own strength while moving through the stretch, they are more helpful for improving functional movements used in everyday life and in sports. In addition, because dynamic-active stretches are movement oriented, these stretches can help generate heat, which can make the muscles more pliable. Finally, evidence suggests that because dynamic-active stretches require muscle activation and contraction, the muscles being stretched are triggered to relax even more than they might during a static-passive stretch, thereby reducing the risk of injury while increasing the functional benefit.

This does not mean you should avoid or minimize static-passive stretching. Just be aware that there appear to be quite a few advantages and benefits to dynamic-active stretching and that you should include these types of stretches as often as is comfortably and conveniently possible for you.

In this book each stretch is labeled as either "passive" or "active." The static stretches include only one photo, whereas the dynamic stretches generally include two photos to show the start and finish positions.

When to Stretch

For many years experts recommended stretching before a workout, activity, or sport. They believed that stretching beforehand reduced the risk of injury and prepped the body for the strenuous effort to come. In fact, before activity was typically the *only* time people stretched, if they stretched at all. Nearly all stretching was static-passive.

In recent years it has become clear that before activity is probably not the best time to stretch. To the surprise of many, studies suggest that people who stretch before they work out might even have a higher rate of injury than those who don't, especially if the stretches are primarily static-passive. Many athletes are consequently stretching less before activity and more following activity, when the soft tissues of their muscles are warm and pliable. Also, as activities such as yoga and Pilates have increased in popularity, many people are now stretching as the primary focus, rather than an ancillary component, of their workout.

This shift in when and how people stretch makes sense. Like all exercise, stretching is designed to create physical stress on the body that requires adaptation that leads to improvement. But if exercises are not done in the best order or at the right time, results can be mixed. For example, runners place stress on their heart and leg muscles when they run. With proper rest, the body recovers from the run, the heart and legs become stronger, and the runner gets fitter over time. However, if the runner attempts to exert maximum effort lifting weights immediately following a hard run, his or her body will probably not respond as beneficially to the weight lifting as it would if the runner had waited a few hours after the run. And, of course, if the runner stops running regularly, and then returns to running as before, the running becomes challenging again until his or her body adapts.

The same principle applies to stretching. When you stretch, you are causing generally nonharmful microscopic damage to soft tissue that ultimately repairs itself, which can lead to greater flexibility over time. Even when a stretch is not painful (it shouldn't be), or when it feels good (the best kind of stretching), it is still physical stress placed on the body to elongate the muscle you are stretching. However, in the moments immediately following a stretch, soft tissue will not be as responsive as it might have been before the stretch. This can make it more difficult for the muscle to produce the power and force required in a workout activity or sport, such as weight lifting or playing soccer. If you stretch your calves, hamstrings, and quads before you play soccer, for instance, you might be reducing the force of your kicks during the game. The normal stress of the soccer game when combined with the stress from the pre-exercise stretches also puts your body at greater risk of injury than if you had not stretched at all before the game.

Instead of stretching before activity, many athletes now warm up their muscles in a different way. A proper warm-up will in fact improve performance and reduce injury risk. The key is to warm up with movements that gradually and progressively simulate the more stressful activity that follows. For example, a 5- to 8-minute power walk or easy jog before a more challenging run likely reduces the risk of injury during the run while improving the runner's speed, pace, and comfort throughout the run. Knee-lift hugs, small kicks, small jumps, shoulder rolls, side steps, and some easy jogging are effective ways to prepare for a soccer match or basketball game.

It is now commonly accepted that the best time to stretch is after activity, when muscle tissue is warm and pliable, or as part of a stand-alone workout that won't be followed by anything that requires powerful muscle contraction or exertion of force. For example, you can stretch at your desk for as little as 5 minutes several times per day, or for as long as 30 to 60 minutes in a yoga class or at home. Instead of stretching aggressively before your weight-training workout or soccer game, warm up lightly in a way that gently introduces your muscles to the upcoming activity.

I know that many of you reading this book have been stretching before your workouts and activities for years, and that what I'm suggesting might be a bit of a shock. In my experience, people who stretch before they work out are attached to doing so and are reluctant to change. In fact, many of my clients, students, and athletes insist they absolutely *do* find that pre-exercise stretching improves their performance and reduces their incidence of injury when they work out or play a sport.

It's hard to argue with what feels right for a particular person. There's no absolute evidence that stretching before working out will automatically increase the risk of injury for every person in every situation. It might not alter your performance at all. But the research that shows it *can* alter performance is persuasive, so at least consider adapting your habits to see if something new works for you. If you do choose to do the stretches or routines in this book before you work out or play sports, make sure to do primarily dynamic-active stretches rather than static-passive ones. This will at least ensure you are increasing your body temperature while you stretch and moving your body in ways that might prepare you for the activity that follows.

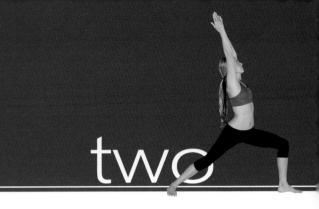

two

Three-Step Stretch System

With 175 stretches, this book probably includes more stretches than you will ever need. Even so, you should approach your stretching in a specific way if you want to achieve optimal results. Whether your goal is to increase your flexibility, get through your day more easily, or improve your performance on the athletic field, you should have a system for linking all of these stretches together and making them work the best they can for you.

Over the years I have developed a stretch system that works incredibly well in my classes and with my clients. Practically speaking, the system is a way of thinking about how to select stretches, how to organize multiple stretches into routines, and how to make sure you aren't stretching too far (or not far enough).

The system includes three simple steps to focus on when stretching, and all you need to remember is this: maximize, minimize, equalize.

Step 1: *Maximize* your range of motion in each stretch.

Step 2: *Minimize* the difference between your passive and active flexibility around each joint and within each muscle group.

Step 3: *Equalize* the range of motion in the left and right sides of the body as well as the front and back sides of the body.

Maximize

Think of range of motion (ROM) in three categories:

1. Tight—below average range of motion.
2. Ideal—normal range of motion.
3. Extraordinary—exceptional range of motion.

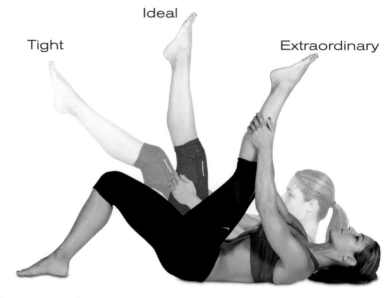

Each photo in this book shows a person with an *ideal* range of motion around a joint(s) for that particular stretch. If you can perform a stretch in this book with the same technique and execution as shown in the photo, you have an ideal range of motion for that stretch. If you are unable to perform the stretch as shown in the photo, you likely have a tight (or limited) range of motion for that stretch. If you can move farther in the direction of the stretch (with good technique) than the photo, you likely have exceptional range of motion for that stretch and around the joint(s).

Your goal should be to maximize your range of motion for each stretch. If you can perform a stretch only with a tight range of motion, your goal should be to practice and perform the stretch working toward an ideal range of motion. If you can perform a stretch with an ideal range of motion (and if you have the time and interest in training harder), your goal is to work toward an extraordinary range of motion.

You might never achieve or move past an ideal range of motion for a particular stretch or around a specific joint, but it is important to measure your progress so that you are working toward at least an ideal range of motion for as many stretches and around as many joints as possible. Of course you must move deeper into a stretch only when you can do so with good technique and without pain; otherwise injury can result.

Remember to mix up your passive and active stretches as you work to maximize your range of motion, and to evaluate and "rank" each stretch and muscle group independent of one another. In other words, it is not ideal to do only passive stretches for the hamstrings. You should also do active stretches for the hamstrings. And just because you exhibit ideal range of motion when performing one particular passive hamstring stretch, that doesn't mean you'll exhibit ideal range of motion during another passive or active hamstring stretch. Spend less time on the stretches and muscle groups in which you exhibit extraordinary range of motion and more time on the stretches and muscle groups in which you exhibit tight range of motion.

Minimize

Assuming you are mixing up your passive and active stretches, your goal is to minimize the difference in range of motion between your passive and active flexibility around each joint and within each muscle group.

For example, if you exhibit ideal range of motion for a passive hamstring stretch but tight range of motion for an active hamstring stretch, you shouldn't push yourself aggressively farther into the passive hamstring stretch (trying to achieve extraordinary range of motion for that stretch) until you have progressed into at least an ideal range of motion for the active hamstring stretch.

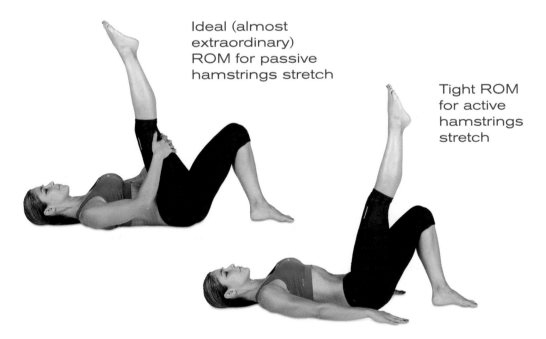

Ideal (almost extraordinary) ROM for passive hamstrings stretch

Tight ROM for active hamstrings stretch

This step ensures that you have the strength and stability around a joint to support the flexibility you are trying to achieve. It also provides a safety net for step 1 by ensuring that, even though you are attempting to maximize your range of motion with each stretch and around each joint, you do not push yourself so far that you become excessively flexible or imbalanced in the type of flexibility you achieve.

Of course you might never have equal passive and active range of motion around each joint and within each muscle group. It makes sense that most of the time you will exhibit greater range of motion with your passive stretches than your active stretches because you have assistance with passive stretches that enables you to push yourself further. That is expected and okay. It is simply important that you do not *increase* the difference in your passive and active range of motion by choosing stretches over time that promote an excessive increase in one over the other.

For instance, I used to have ideal range of motion in my chest and shoulder joint when I stretched passively. But when I did active stretches for my chest and shoulder joint, it was clear that I used to be tight. I simply could not move myself actively into positions that stretched my chest and shoulder joint nearly as well as I could perform similar passive stretches for the same area. This was likely because my back muscles (which must contract to stretch my chest and shoulder joint in an active stretch) were not as strong as my chest was flexible. So I was easily able to *leverage* myself into an ideal range of motion, but I couldn't *move* myself into an ideal range of motion.

I could have simply pushed myself to go from ideal passive flexibility to extraordinary passive flexibility in my chest and shoulder joint, ignoring the fact that my active flexibility in these areas was less than ideal. But instead I worked to improve my active range of motion in the chest and shoulder joint. I did more active chest and shoulder joint stretches and moved my active range of motion in these areas closer to ideal *before* pushing myself to an extraordinary range of motion with the passive stretches.

This accomplished two things. First, because my upper back muscles had to engage to perform active stretches for my chest and shoulder joint, my upper back got stronger. I saw a noticeable difference in my posture and could feel the strength and stability in my shoulder joint improve. Second, I could more easily improve my passive flexibility in my chest and shoulder joint because of the neuromuscular stimulus (discussed later in this chapter) provided by the additional active stretching.

By training with this second step in mind, I have achieved extraordinary passive *and* active flexibility in my chest and shoulder joint, and this area of my body is now stronger, more flexible, and less prone to injury.

Step 2 is important. For many people, it is easy to select the perfect passive stretches for a variety of muscle groups that enables them to exhibit ideal range of motion. And it is easy to simply work to improve your range of motion in the passive stretches in which you already have this ideal range of motion.

However, improvements in flexibility should be achieved holistically, not only within stretches, muscles groups, and joint areas where you are already ideal. Working to make your passive and active range of motion comparable across multiple muscle groups and stretches will provide amazing benefits, helping you reduce your risk of injury while making you stronger and more flexible.

Equalize

When you stretch, you will likely notice that the left and right sides of your body do not respond the same. You will also notice differences when you compare the front and back sides of your body. For example, in some cases you will be able to perform a stretch with ideal range of motion on your right side, but you'll exhibit tight range of motion on your left side with the same stretch. Or you might find that you are extraordinarily flexible through your quadriceps (front of the body) but not as flexible through your hamstrings (back of the body). This is normal. Nearly everyone has some degree of muscular imbalance. Our third step involves working to improve these imbalances through deliberate and thoughtful adjustments in the type (and amount) of specific stretches you do, and in how intensely you do them.

If you notice, for example, that your chest and front shoulder are tight, but your upper back and rear shoulders are ideal or extraordinarily flexible, you should organize your stretch routines to include more stretches for your chest and front shoulder than for your upper back and rear shoulder. This does not mean ignoring your upper back and rear shoulders. Just make sure your ratio of stretches favors your chest and front shoulder. You might do three chest and front shoulder stretches for every one upper back and rear shoulder stretch. Over time, you'll begin to notice your range of motion in these two opposing areas have become closer to equal.

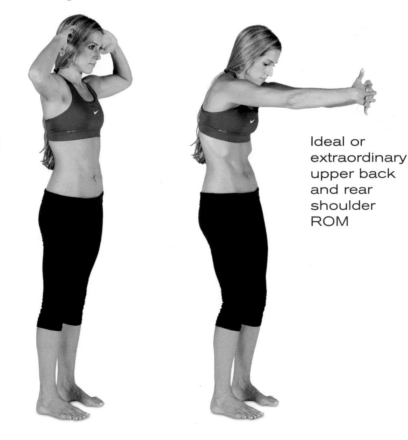

Tight chest and front shoulder ROM

Ideal or extraordinary upper back and rear shoulder ROM

Say you are performing a gluteal stretch, and you notice extraordinary range of motion in your right hip but tight range of motion in your left hip. You should probably ease up on the intensity of the right hip stretch and be slightly more aggressive in your left hip stretch. Over time, you'll notice the left hip moves closer to ideal, and the right hip moves closer to ideal, and they will be more similar to each other in terms of range of motion.

This effort to equalize the range of motion in the front and back sides of the body as well as in the left and right sides of the body will help improve your everyday movement patterns, reduce your risk of movement-based injury, minimize the chances of back pain, and improve your athletic ability.

I find that I must discipline myself to watch this third step carefully. I tend to emphasize the side of the body in which I am more flexible because I feel more successful on that side. And, of course, stretching the more flexible side often *feels* better than stretching the tighter side. However, adjusting the stretches you do and the intensity with which you do them to promote equalization is the smart thing to do; this will help give you the well-rounded results you want and need from your flexibility training.

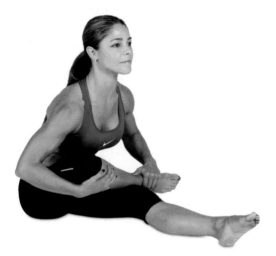

Extraordinary right hip ROM

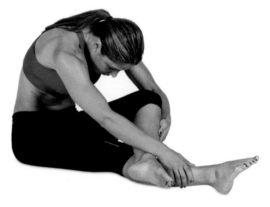

Tight left hip ROM

Breathing

Both scientific research and anecdotal evidence suggest that thoughtful and deliberate breathing patterns can enhance or improve nervous system responses, improve respiratory and cardiovascular function, decrease effects of stress, and improve physical and mental health. But does a style or pattern of breathing improve or enhance the benefit of an individual stretch or stretching routine? If you have participated in an authentic yoga class, you know that specific breathing patterns are taught as a way to support and enhance the benefit of the poses and sequences (as well as to stimulate what yogis consider to be the "life force" or central energy of the body). And most people who work out regularly have at some point been instructed on proper breathing patterns for various exercises to improve the result and minimize the chances of hyperventilating or feeling light-headed.

But it is also true that many athletes and fitness enthusiasts have improved their flexibility through stretching without using any particular style or pattern of breathing. It's likely that you too can benefit from the stretches in this book without having to worry much about how and when you breathe while performing the stretches. That said, I have personally seen most of my students and clients generally feel better and experience greater success when they are at least mindful about their breathing when they stretch. At the bare minimum, I encourage them to exhale as they move into a passive stretch, and to breathe deeply and evenly while holding a static-passive stretch. I also encourage them to inhale and exhale in a rhythmic pattern that matches the movement of any dynamic stretches. I have found that incorporating these simple breathing patterns creates a greater connection to the stretch and helps the muscles, joints, and body relax and respond with greater sensitivity.

I have provided simple breathing cues with every stretch description. If comfortable doing so, incorporate these breathing patterns as you execute each stretch. Many of you will already have an established style or pattern of breathing you use when stretching that you have developed on your own or learned from a coach or yoga instructor. If this breathing pattern feels right to you, stick with it. If the pattern does not enhance your experience with these stretches, try my suggestions.

As you become more advanced with your flexibility training, you'll likely find that deep, controlled, rhythmic, purposeful, and relaxed breathing becomes a natural part of your stretching routine. You might also find that regularly using this type of breathing helps you feel calmer and more clearheaded.

FRONT

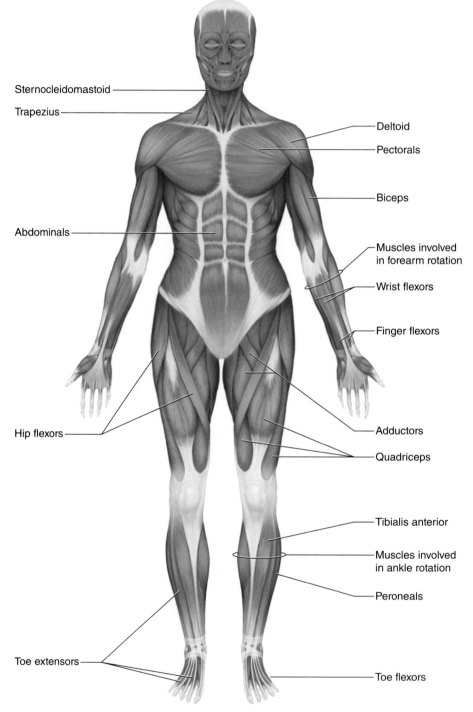

Sternocleidomastoid

Trapezius

Deltoid

Pectorals

Biceps

Abdominals

Muscles involved
in forearm rotation

Wrist flexors

Finger flexors

Hip flexors

Adductors

Quadriceps

Tibialis anterior

Muscles involved
in ankle rotation

Peroneals

Toe extensors

Toe flexors

Use this full-body muscle diagram to identify targeted muscle groups.

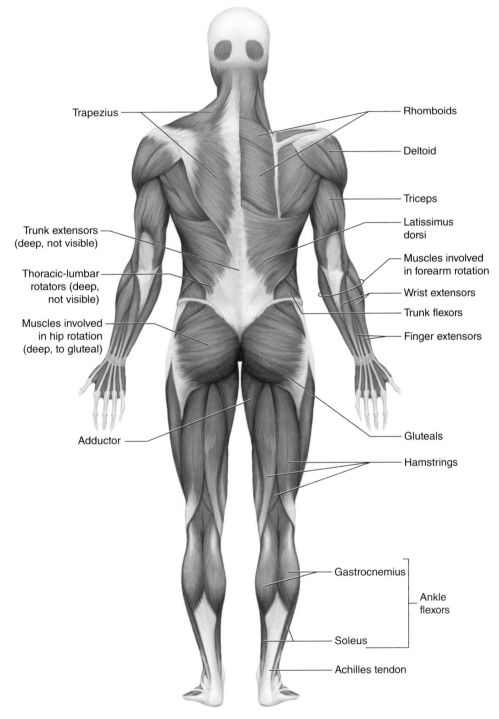

Trapezius

Rhomboids

Deltoid

Triceps

Latissimus dorsi

Trunk extensors (deep, not visible)

Muscles involved in forearm rotation

Thoracic-lumbar rotators (deep, not visible)

Wrist extensors

Trunk flexors

Muscles involved in hip rotation (deep, to gluteal)

Finger extensors

Adductor

Gluteals

Hamstrings

Gastrocnemius

Ankle flexors

Soleus

Achilles tendon

Use this full-body muscle diagram to identify targeted muscle groups.

part II

Regions of Flexibility

Neck, Shoulders, Arms, and Hands

Chest, Back, and Abdominals

Glutes, Hips, and Inner Thighs

Quadriceps and Hamstrings

Calves, Shins, and Feet

Multiregion Stretches

Sport Mobility Stretches

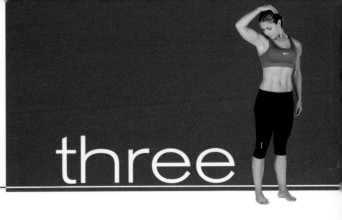

three

Neck, Shoulders, Arms, and Hands

In this chapter we'll focus on stretching the muscles that support the head and control the movement of the arms and hands. Don't be surprised if you discover you are tighter than you expect when performing some of these stretches. These muscles, though important for total body function, are often overlooked in many people's flexibility routines.

Neck

I think you'll be pleasantly surprised to discover how relaxing and rewarding it is to do the neck stretches. These stretches help with movements that contribute to everyday tasks you might take for granted, such as looking over your shoulder to change lanes on the freeway or looking up to catch a ball. The stretches also reduce headaches caused by tension and provide relief for a sore neck that can come from sleeping in an airplane seat or uncomfortable bed.

Head Tilt

Sternocleidomastoid, trapezius

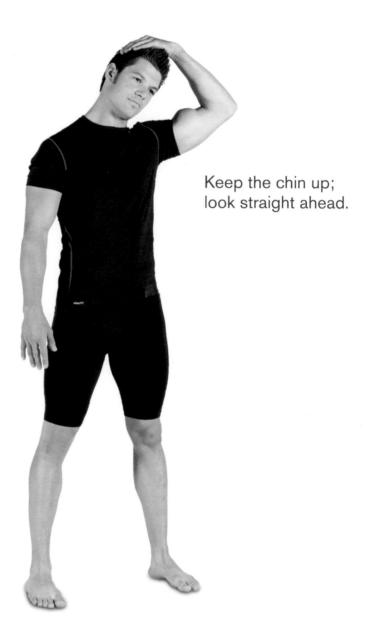

Keep the chin up;
look straight ahead.

- Stand or sit tall. Lower one ear toward the shoulder. Gently pull down from the opposite side of the head.
- Hold the stretch for 10 to 30 seconds.
- Repeat on the other side.

 Exhale deeply while moving into the farthest point of the stretch; then breathe evenly while holding the stretch.

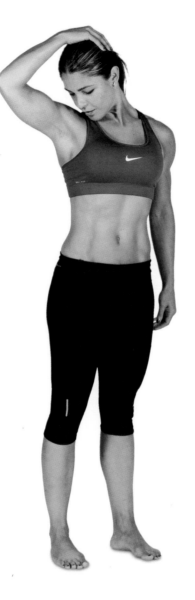

Don't round
the spine.

- Stand or sit tall. Drop the chin diagonally toward the armpit as far as comfortably possible. Place one hand on the back of the head and pull gently toward the armpit.
- Hold the stretch for 10 to 30 seconds.
- Repeat on the other side.

breathe **Exhale deeply while moving into the farthest point of the stretch; then breathe evenly while holding the stretch.**

Head Turn

Sternocleidomastoid, trapezius

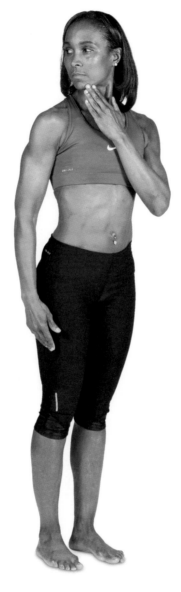

Keep the chin up.

- Stand or sit tall. Turn the head as far to one side as comfortably possible.
- Place one hand on the side of the chin and gently push.
- Hold the stretch for 10 to 30 seconds.

breathe **Exhale deeply while moving into the farthest point of the stretch; then breathe evenly while holding the stretch.**

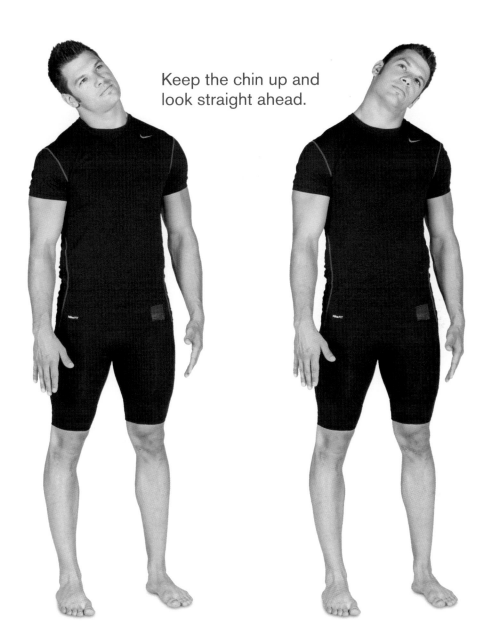

Keep the chin up and look straight ahead.

- Stand or sit tall.
- Lower one ear toward the shoulder while lifting the opposite ear toward the ceiling.
- Release the stretch by returning the head to neutral position. Repeat on the other side.
- Each repetition of the sequence should take 1 to 3 seconds. Repeat as a continuous, controlled, fluid sequence 10 to 12 times.

breathe **Exhale while lowering the ear toward the shoulder; inhale each time the stretch is released.**

25

Dynamic Head Turn
Sternocleidomastoid, trapezius

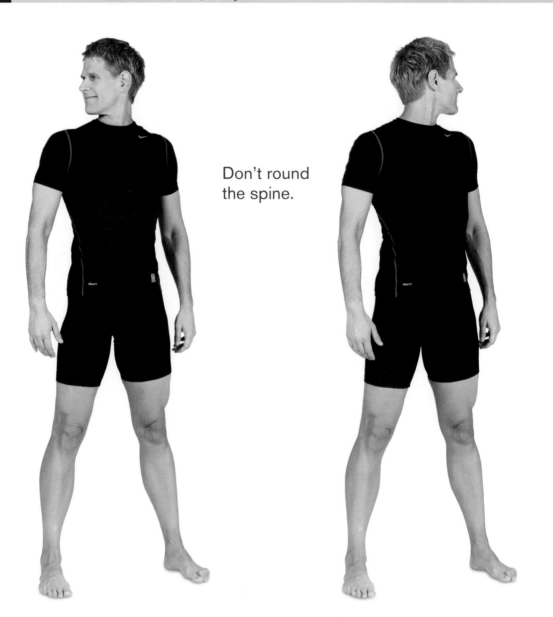

Don't round
the spine.

- Stand or sit tall.
- Turn the head as far to one side as comfortably possible.
- Release the stretch by returning the head to neutral position.
- Repeat on the other side.
- Each repetition of the sequence should take 1 to 3 seconds. Repeat as a continuous, controlled, fluid sequence 10 to 12 times.

breathe **Exhale while turning the head to one side; inhale each time the stretch is released.**

Dynamic Diagonal Chin Drop

Sternocleidomastoid, trapezius

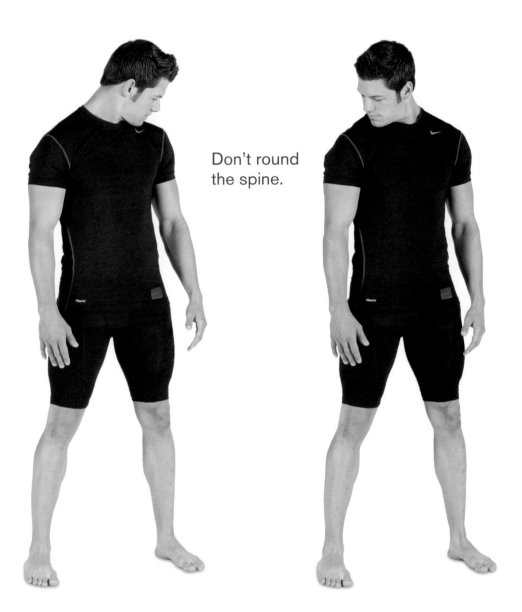

Don't round
the spine.

- ▌ Stand or sit tall.
- ▌ Drop the chin diagonally toward the armpit as far as comfortably possible while lifting the back of the head toward the ceiling.
- ▌ Release the stretch by lifting the head to neutral position.
- ▌ Repeat on the other side.
- ▌ Each repetition of the sequence should take 1 to 3 seconds. Repeat as a continuous, controlled, fluid sequence 10 to 12 times.

breathe **Exhale while dropping the chin toward the armpit; inhale each time the stretch is released.**

Reach Behind Head Tilt

Trapezius

Stand tall; look straight ahead.

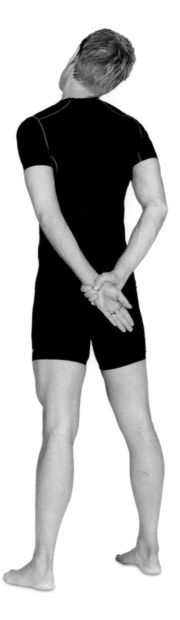

- Stand with the feet apart and arms next to the body. Slowly drop the head to one side. Reach behind and pull down on the wrist of the opposite arm.
- Hold the stretch for 10 to 30 seconds.
- Repeat on the other side.

breathe **Exhale deeply while moving into the farthest point of the stretch; then breathe evenly while holding the stretch.**

28

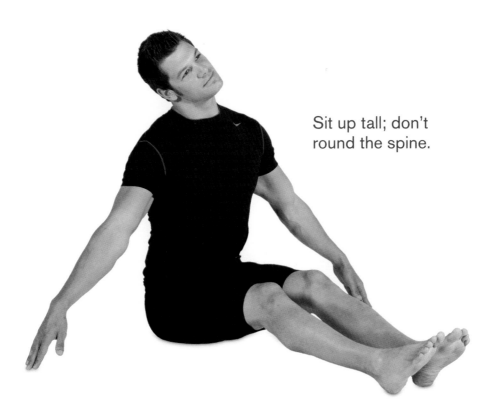

Sit up tall; don't round the spine.

- Sit with the legs in front of the body and the knees slightly bent.
- Reach out as far as possible to both sides, touching the floor; slowly drop the head to one side.
- Hold the stretch for 10 to 30 seconds.
- Repeat on the other side.

 Exhale deeply while moving into the farthest point of the stretch; then breathe evenly while holding the stretch.

Dynamic Chin Drop

Trapezius

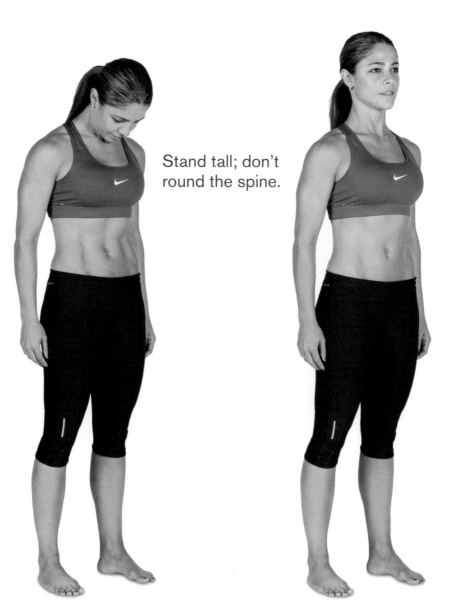

Stand tall; don't round the spine.

- Stand with the feet apart and the arms alongside the body.
- Slowly drop the head forward and gently bring the chin closer to the chest by contracting the muscles in the front of the neck.
- Release the stretch by lifting the head to neutral position.
- Each repetition of the sequence should take 1 to 3 seconds. Repeat as a continuous, controlled, fluid sequence 10 to 12 times.

breathe **Exhale while dropping the head forward; inhale each time the stretch is released.**

Shoulders

The major muscles that control the movement of the shoulders are the trapezius (the kite-shaped muscle on the back) and the deltoids, which cover the front, top, and rear of the shoulder joint. Stretching these muscles improves your posture and makes it easier to reach up with your arms or reach behind you. Like the neck stretches, these stretches reduce headaches caused by tension and provide relief for a sore neck.

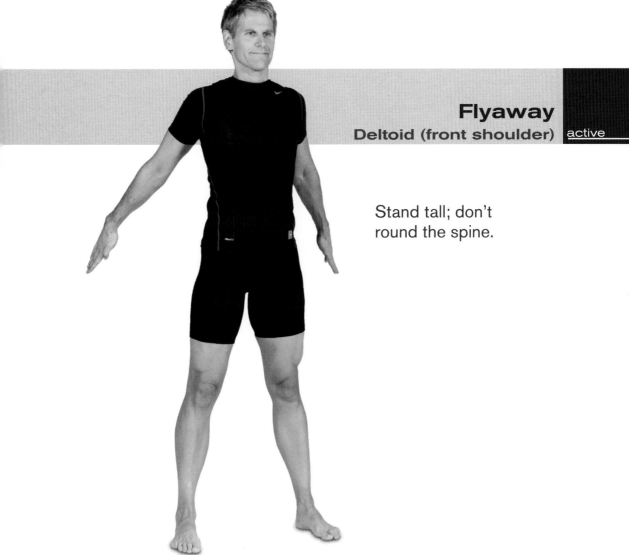

Flyaway
Deltoid (front shoulder) active

Stand tall; don't round the spine.

- ❚ Stand with the feet apart. Lift the arms out to the side of the body below shoulder height, palms facing down.
- ❚ Reach behind as far as comfortably possible, keeping the elbows straight.
- ❚ Hold the stretch for 10 to 30 seconds.

breathe **Exhale deeply while moving into the farthest point of the stretch; then breathe evenly while holding the stretch.**

Reach Behind and Open

Deltoid (front shoulder)

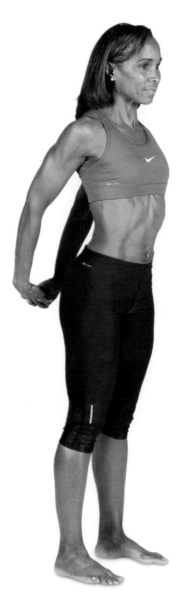

Stand tall;
don't round
the spine.

- ▌ Stand with the feet shoulder-width apart.
- ▌ Clasp the hands together in the small of the back and lift the arms upward.
- ▌ Hold the stretch for 10 to 30 seconds.

breathe **Exhale deeply while moving into the farthest point of the stretch; then breathe evenly while holding the stretch.**

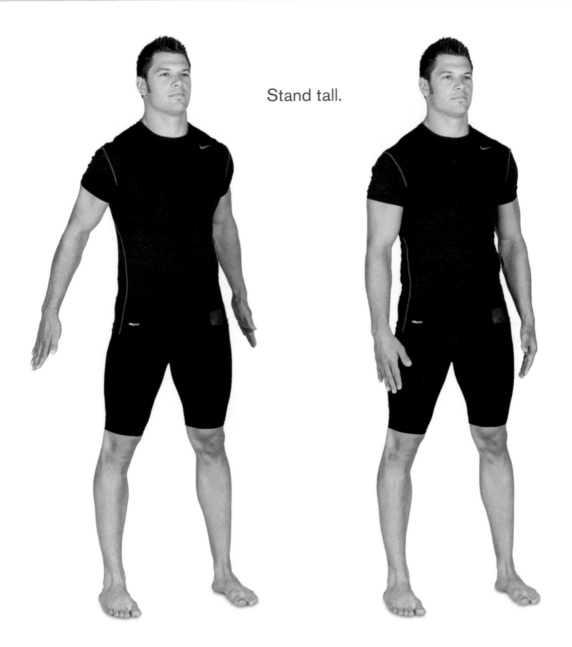

Stand tall.

- Stand with the feet apart.
- Lift the arms a few inches (several centimeters) away from the hips; slowly lift the arms behind the body.
- Release the stretch by returning the arms to the side of the body.
- Each repetition of the sequence should take 1 to 3 seconds. Repeat as a continuous, controlled, fluid sequence 10 to 12 times.

 Exhale while lifting the arms behind the body; inhale each time the stretch is released.

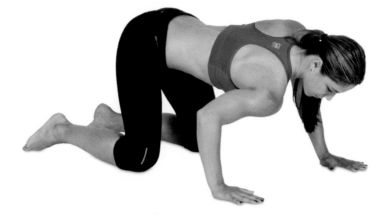

Don't arch the back.

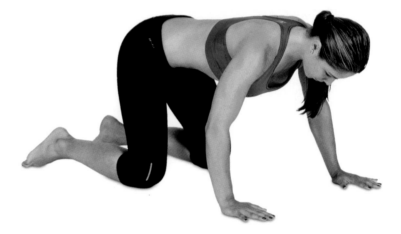

- Kneel on the floor on the hands and the knees.
- Gently push one shoulder toward the floor.
- Release the stretch by moving the shoulder level with the opposite shoulder.
- Repeat on the other side.
- Each repetition of the sequence should take 1 to 3 seconds. Repeat as a continuous, controlled, fluid sequence 10 to 12 times.

 Exhale while pushing the shoulder toward the floor; inhale each time the stretch is released.

Sit up tall; keep
the chin lifted.

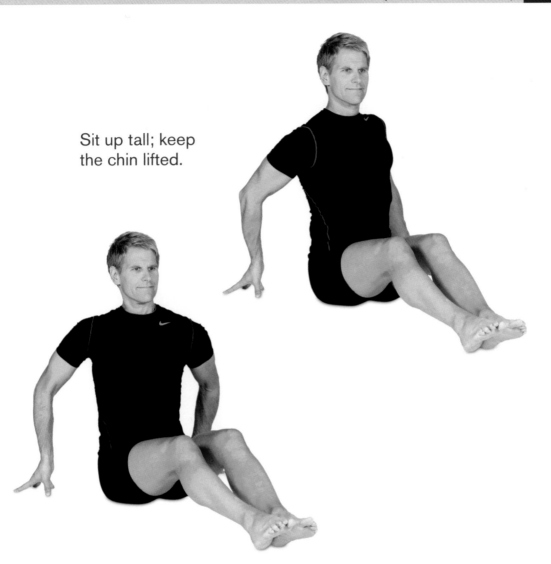

- ▌ Sit down; place both legs straight in front with the knees slightly bent.
- ▌ Place the hands on the floor behind the body and press one shoulder toward the feet.
- ▌ Release the stretch by moving the shoulder away from the feet and level with the opposite shoulder.
- ▌ Repeat on the other side.
- ▌ Each repetition of the sequence should take 1 to 3 seconds. Repeat as a continuous, controlled, fluid sequence 10 to 12 times.

breathe

Exhale while pressing the shoulder toward the feet; inhale each time the stretch is released.

Dynamic Faucet Hands
Deltoid (rotator cuff)

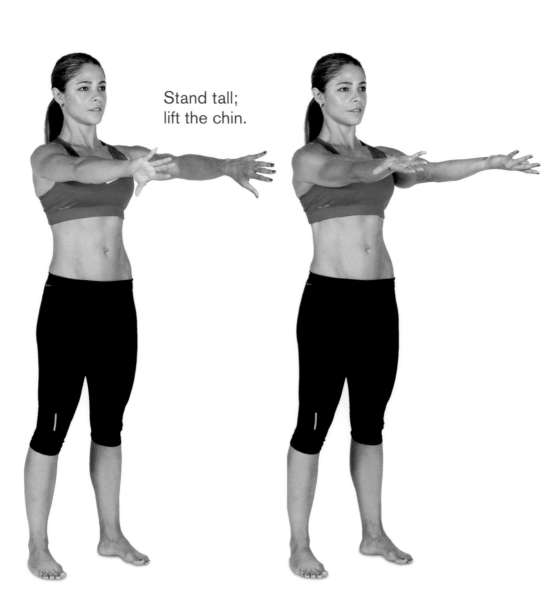

Stand tall;
lift the chin.

- Stand with the arms in front of the body at shoulder height, the palms facing each other.
- Twist the hands inward as far as comfortably possible (similar to turning faucets).
- Twist the hands in the opposite direction.
- Each repetition of the sequence should take 1 to 3 seconds. Repeat as a continuous, controlled, fluid sequence 10 to 12 times.

breathe **Breathe evenly while performing the sequence.**

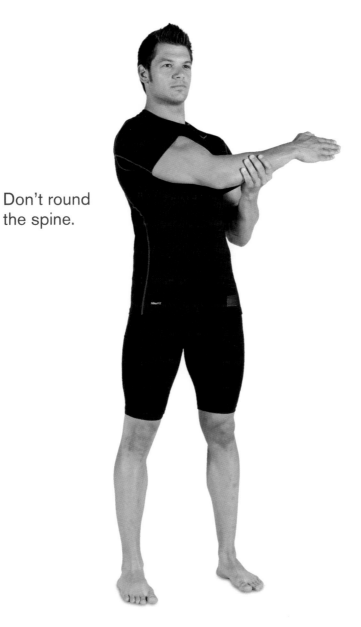

Don't round
the spine.

▮ Stand with the feet shoulder-width apart. Bring one arm directly across the body at chest height and hold it in place with the opposite arm.

▮ Hold the stretch for 10 to 30 seconds.

▮ Repeat the stretch with the other arm.

 Exhale deeply while moving into the farthest point of the stretch; then breathe evenly while holding the stretch.

Dynamic Arm Across
Deltoid (rear shoulder)

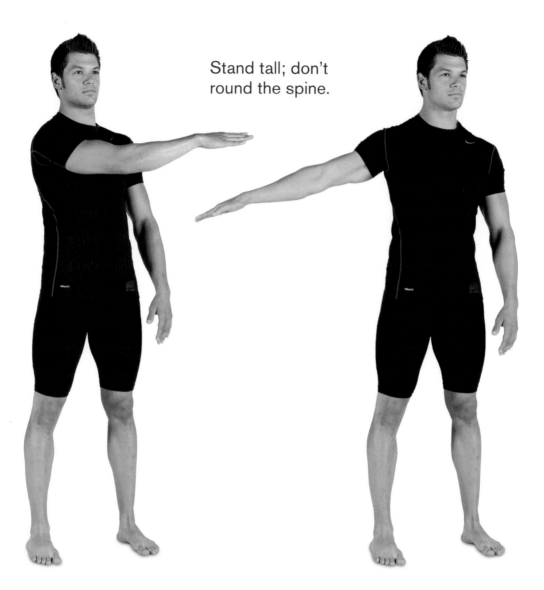

Stand tall; don't round the spine.

- Stand with the feet apart.
- Bring one arm across the body at chest height as far as comfortably possible.
- Release the stretch by bringing the arm out to the side of the body at chest height.
- Each repetition of the sequence should take 1 to 3 seconds. Repeat as a continuous, controlled, fluid sequence 10 to 12 times.
- Repeat the stretch with the other arm.

breathe **Exhale while bringing the arm across the body; inhale each time the stretch is released.**

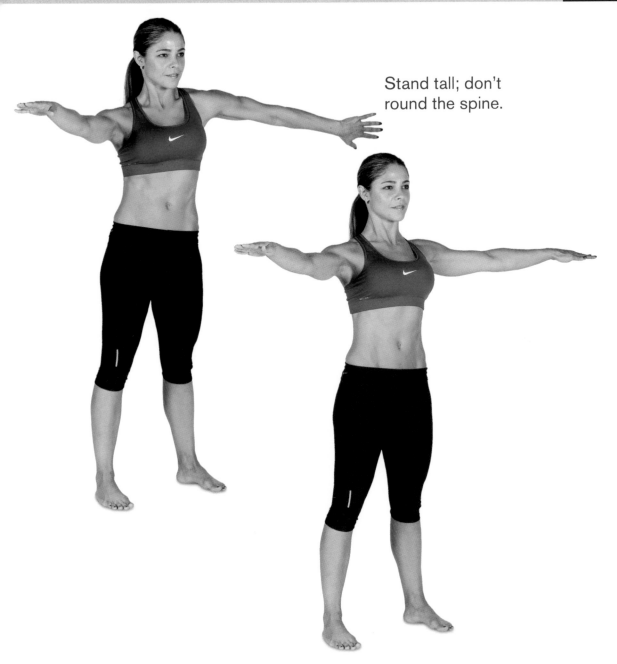

Stand tall; don't round the spine.

- Stand with the feet shoulder-width apart and the arms lifted to shoulder height.
- Roll one shoulder toward the feet.
- Release the stretch by rolling the shoulder back to a neutral position.
- Each repetition of the sequence should take 1 to 3 seconds. Repeat as a continuous, controlled, fluid sequence 10 to 12 times on both sides of the body.

 breathe **Exhale while rolling the shoulder toward the feet; inhale each time the stretch is released.**

Arms

We're constantly pushing, pulling, lifting, and lowering things all day. These stretches help lengthen and strengthen the muscles used for these tasks and make it easier to perform them throughout the day.

Pronated Reach Back and Turn

passive **Biceps**

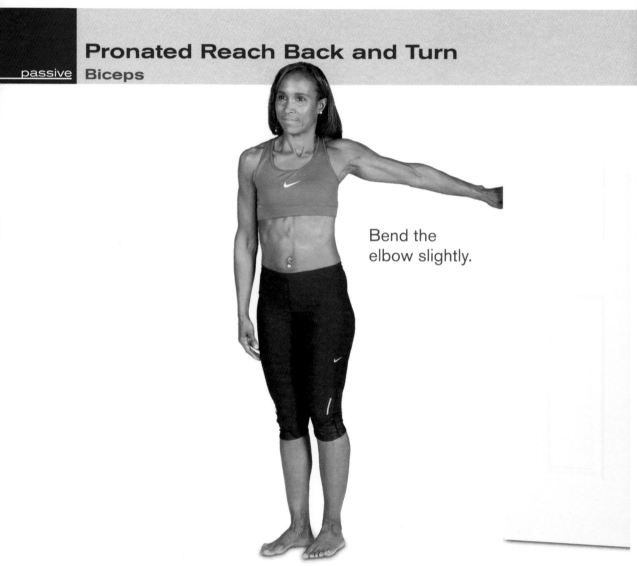

Bend the elbow slightly.

- Stand and raise one arm to the side at shoulder height. Place the back of the hand (thumb down) against a stationary object, such as a wall or door. Slowly rotate the upper body away from the hand.
- Hold the stretch for 10 to 30 seconds.
- Repeat the stretch with the other arm.

 breathe **Exhale deeply while moving into the farthest point of the stretch; then breathe evenly while holding the stretch.**

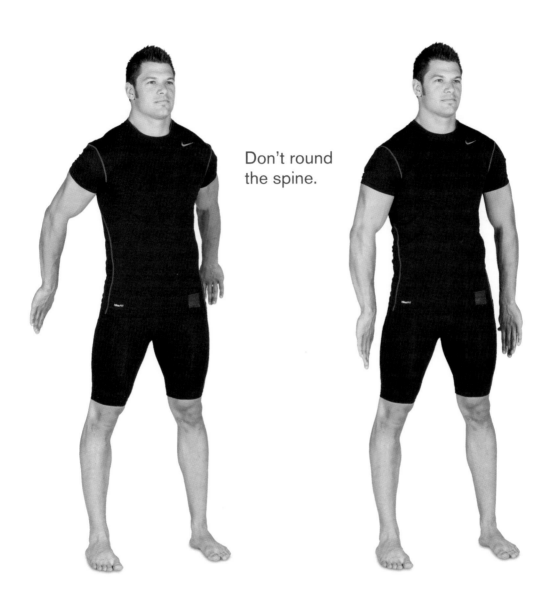

Don't round
the spine.

- Stand with the hands at the sides and the palms facing back.
- Lift the arms behind the body and toward the ceiling while twisting the palms outward.
- Release the stretch by lowering the arms to the sides of the body.
- Each repetition of the sequence should take 1 to 3 seconds. Repeat as a continuous, controlled, fluid sequence 10 to 12 times.

 Exhale while lifting the arms behind the body and inhale each time the stretch is released.

Elbow Bend and Push

Triceps

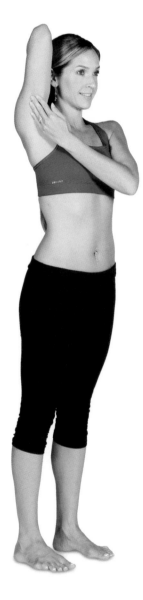

Keep the
chin up.

- Stand or sit tall. Lift one arm above the head. Bend the elbow and place the hand between the shoulder blades. Use the other hand to gently push the elbow back.
- Hold the stretch for 10 to 30 seconds.
- Repeat the stretch with the other arm.

breathe **Exhale deeply while moving into the farthest point of the stretch; then breathe evenly while holding the stretch.**

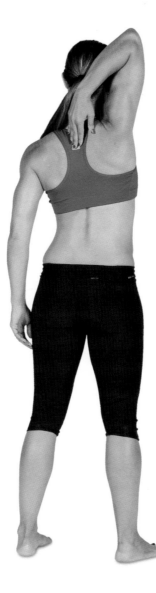

Keep the
chin up.

- Stand or sit tall. Lift one arm above the head. Bend the elbow and place the hand between the shoulder blades as far down as comfortably possible.
- Hold the stretch for 10 to 30 seconds.
- Repeat the stretch with the other arm.

breathe

Exhale deeply while moving into the farthest point of the stretch; then breathe evenly while holding the stretch.

Kneeling Elbow Push
Triceps

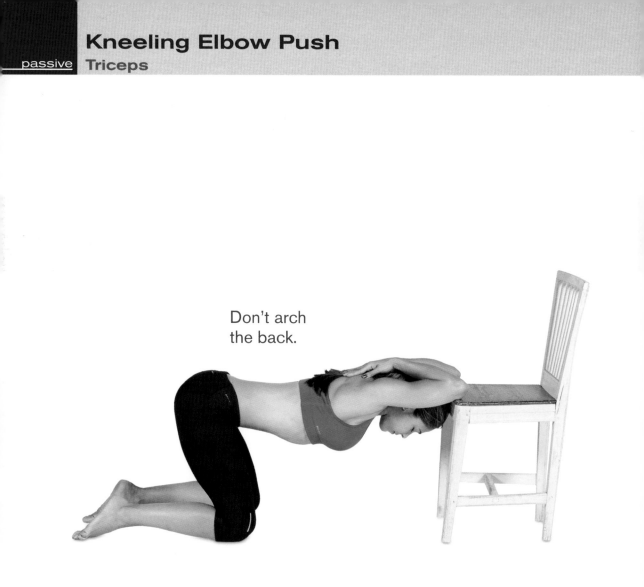

Don't arch
the back.

- Kneel in front of a chair or platform. Place both hands on the back of the shoulder. Anchor the elbows on the chair or platform. Lean forward at the hips and bring the chest toward the floor.
- Hold the stretch for 10 to 30 seconds.

breathe **Exhale deeply while moving into the farthest point of the stretch; then breathe evenly while holding the stretch.**

Hands

We use our forearms, wrists, and fingers to perform many repetitive tasks, such as typing on a keyboard, gripping a steering wheel, or texting on a cell phone. The stretches in this section increase mobility in the forearms, wrists, and fingers and help reverse the mechanical stress associated with hand and forearm overuse injuries.

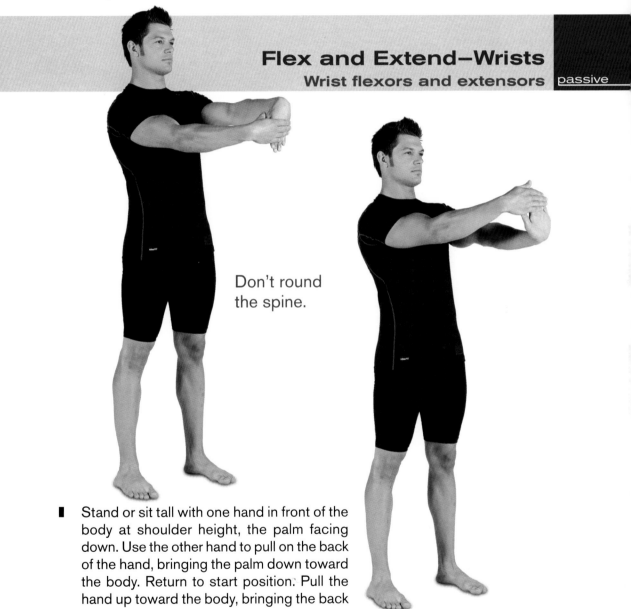

Flex and Extend—Wrists
Wrist flexors and extensors | passive

Don't round
the spine.

- ▌ Stand or sit tall with one hand in front of the body at shoulder height, the palm facing down. Use the other hand to pull on the back of the hand, bringing the palm down toward the body. Return to start position. Pull the hand up toward the body, bringing the back of the hand up.
- ▌ Hold each stretch for 10 to 30 seconds.
- ▌ Repeat the stretch with the other hand.

 breathe   **Exhale deeply while moving into the farthest point of the stretch; then breathe evenly while holding the stretch.**

Dynamic Flex and Extend—Wrists
Wrist flexors and extensors

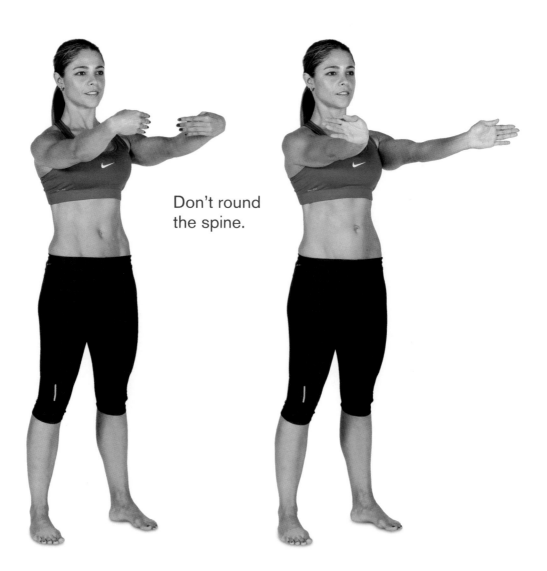

Don't round
the spine.

- Stand or sit with the arms held out in front at shoulder height and the palms facing each other.
- Flex the wrists, turning the palms toward the body.
- Extend the wrists, turning the palms away from the body.
- Each repetition of the sequence should take 1 to 3 seconds. Repeat as a continuous, controlled, fluid sequence 10 to 12 times.

breathe   **Breathe evenly while performing the sequence.**

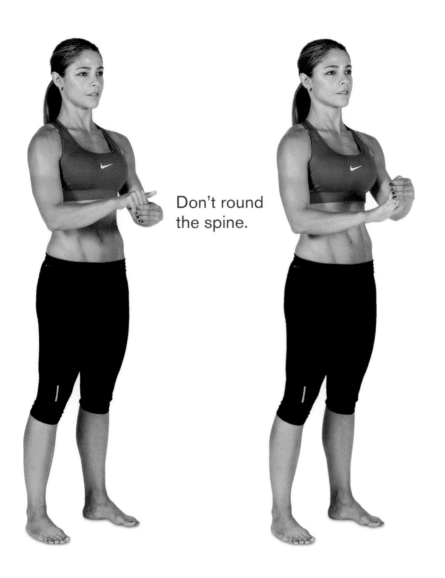

Don't round
the spine.

- Stand or sit; use one hand to first push down and then pull back on the fingers of the other hand.
- Hold each stretch for 10 to 30 seconds in both positions.
- Repeat the stretches with the other hand.

breathe **Exhale deeply while moving into the farthest point of the stretch; then breathe evenly while holding the stretch.**

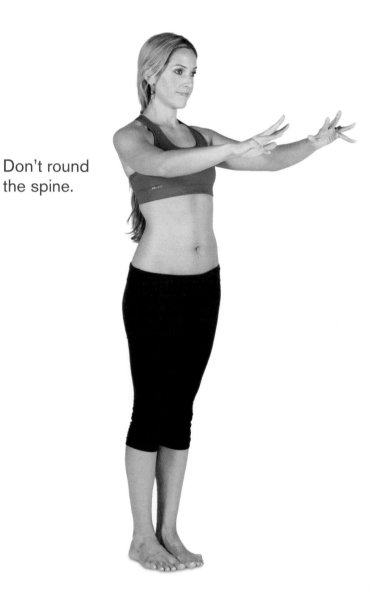

Don't round
the spine.

▮ Stand or sit with the arms held out in front of the body. Wiggle the fingers in all directions as if playing the piano.

▮ Repeat as a continuous, controlled, fluid sequence 10 to 30 seconds.

breathe **Breathe evenly while performing the sequence.**

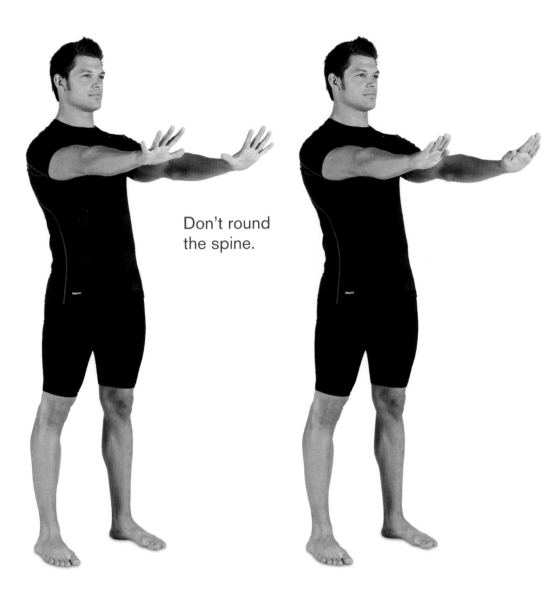

Don't round
the spine.

- Stand or sit with the arms held out in front of the body, the palms facing away.
- Spread the fingers as far apart as comfortably possible.
- Release the stretch by bringing the fingers together.
- Each repetition of the sequence should take 1 to 3 seconds. Repeat as a continuous, controlled, fluid sequence 10 to 12 times.

breathe **Breathe evenly while performing the sequence.**

Dynamic Ball Wrist Rolls
Wrist flexors and extensors

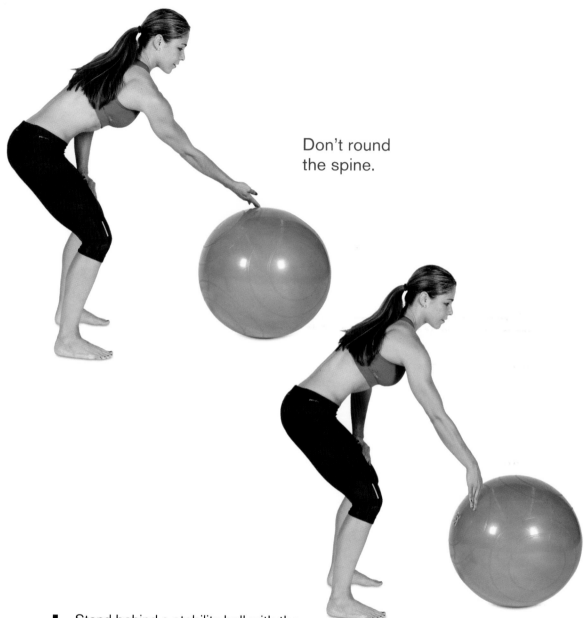

Don't round
the spine.

- Stand behind a stability ball with the knees bent and one hand placed on top of the ball.
- Move the hand in a clockwise motion, rotating the ball in a circle.
- Move the hand in a counterclockwise motion, rotating the ball in a circle.
- Each repetition of the sequence should take 1 to 3 seconds. Repeat as a continuous, controlled, fluid sequence 10 to 12 times.
- Repeat the movements with the other hand.

breathe **Breathe evenly while performing the sequence.**

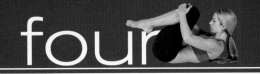

four

Chest, Back, and Abdominals

This chapter focuses on the muscles in the torso that work together to protect and stabilize the spine and strengthen your core. Muscle imbalance in this region of the body can lead to poor posture and back pain, so these muscles need to be stretched frequently with the three-step system in mind.

Chest

If you're like most people, the muscles in your chest are tighter than the muscles in your back. This is because you spend a good part of the day with your shoulders rounded forward working at your desk, driving your car, carrying things, or reaching forward to pick things up. By performing stretches for the chest (especially dynamic-active stretches), you can create a better balance between chest flexibility and back strength.

Kneeling Reach
Pectorals

Don't sit too heavily
on the feet.

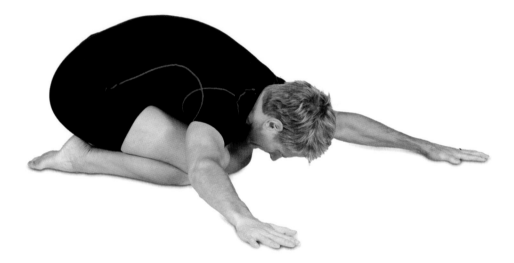

- ▌ Kneeling on the floor, extend the arms directly out in front of the body while pushing the chest down toward the floor.
- ▌ Hold each stretch for 10 to 30 seconds.

breathe **Exhale deeply while moving into the farthest point of the stretch; then breathe evenly while holding the stretch.**

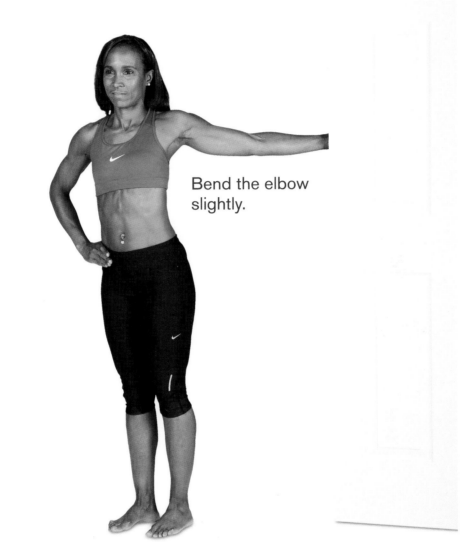

Bend the elbow
slightly.

▌ Stand and raise one arm to the side at shoulder height. Hold onto a stationary
  object, such as a door or cabinet. Slowly rotate the upper body away from
  the hand.

▌ Hold the stretch for 10 to 30 seconds.

▌ Repeat the movements using the other arm.

 **Exhale deeply while moving into the farthest point of the
stretch; then breathe evenly while holding the stretch.**

Chest Expansion
Pectorals

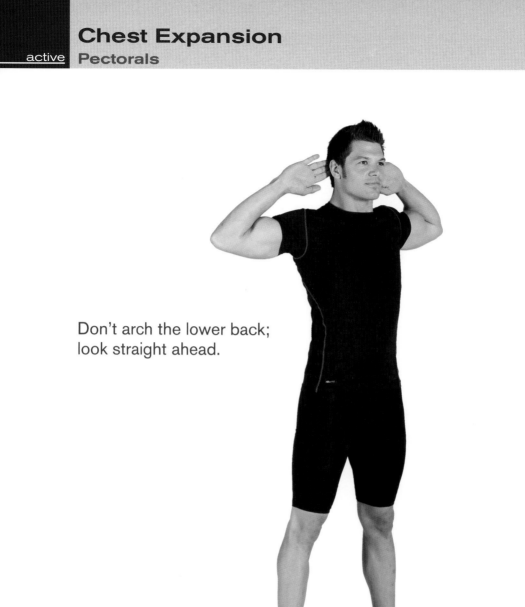

Don't arch the lower back;
look straight ahead.

- Hold the elbows at shoulder height with the fingers near the ears. Squeeze the shoulder blades together and pull the elbows back.
- Hold the stretch for 10 to 30 seconds.

 Exhale deeply while moving into the farthest point of the stretch; then breathe evenly while holding the stretch.

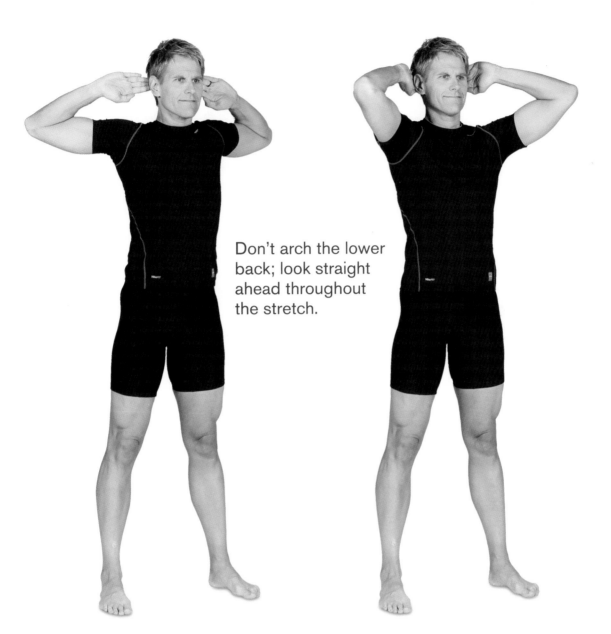

Don't arch the lower back; look straight ahead throughout the stretch.

- Hold the elbows at shoulder height with the fingers near the ears.
- Squeeze the shoulder blades together and pull the elbows back.
- Release the stretch by bringing the elbows in front of the ears.
- Each repetition of the sequence should take 1 to 3 seconds. Repeat as a continuous, controlled, fluid sequence 10 to 12 times.

breathe **Exhale while squeezing the shoulder blades together; inhale each time the stretch is released.**

Dynamic Reach Back and Turn
Pectorals

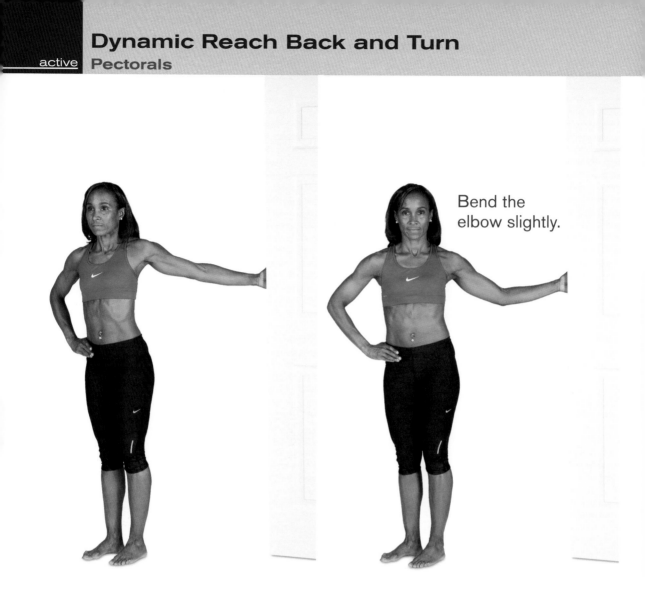

Bend the elbow slightly.

- Stand and raise one arm to the side at shoulder height. Hold onto a stationary object, such as a door or cabinet.
- Slowly turn the upper body away from the hand, squeezing the shoulder blades together.
- Release the stretch by returning the upper body to the start position.
- Repeat the movements with the other arm.
- Each repetition of the sequence should take 1 to 3 seconds. Repeat as a continuous, controlled, fluid sequence 10 to 12 times.

breathe **Exhale while turning the upper body away from the hand; inhale each time the stretch is released.**

Don't extend beyond the point that's comfortable for the lower back.

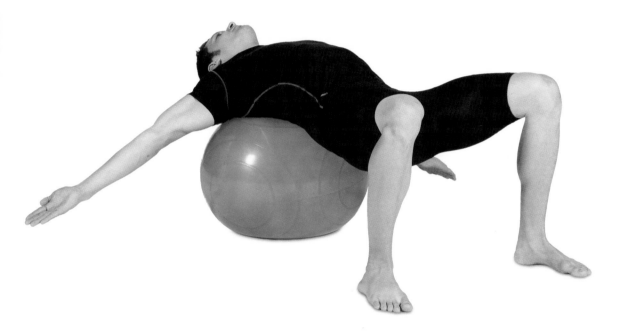

▮ Place the middle back on the center of a stability ball with the feet on the floor and the knees bent. Extending the arms out to the sides of the body, reach as far away from the body as comfortably possible.

▮ Hold the stretch for 10 to 30 seconds.

Exhale deeply while moving into the farthest point of the stretch; then breathe evenly while holding the stretch.

Back

Back injuries are the second most common medical complaint in the United States (headaches are the first). Although there's no one reason for back pain or injury, tightness and reduced mobility in the back are significant contributing factors. The stretches described here will improve mobility in the spine, deliver oxygen to the discs in the back, and reduce overall muscle tension that can lead to discomfort.

Scoop

passive **Rhomboids**

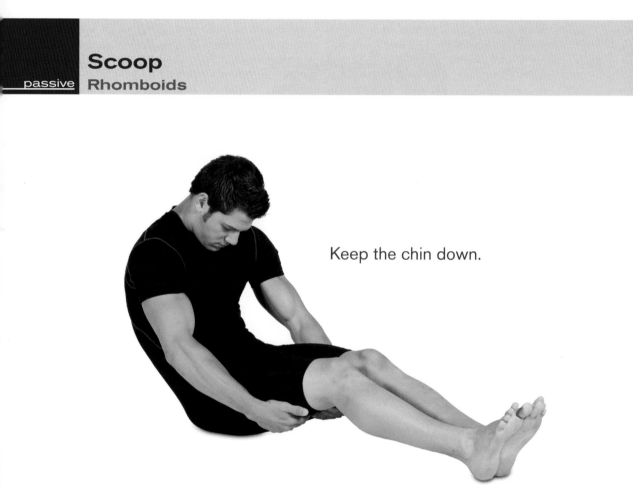

Keep the chin down.

- Sitting on the floor, extend the legs straight in front with the knees slightly bent. Lean forward, reach for the back of the thighs, and round the back.
- Hold the stretch for 10 to 30 seconds.

breathe **Exhale deeply while moving into the farthest point of the stretch; then breathe evenly while holding the stretch.**

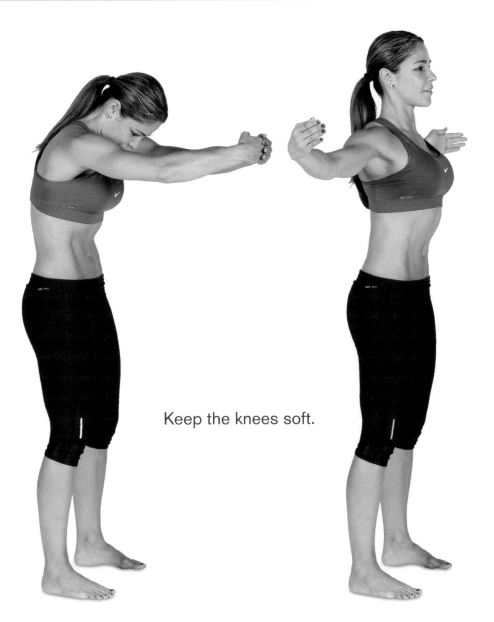

Keep the knees soft.

- Stand with the feet shoulder-width apart.
- Round the shoulders and reach forward with elbows bent. Clasp the hands together. Drop the chin toward the chest. Squeeze the chest to stretch the middle back.
- Release the stretch by unlocking the hands; bring the arms out to the sides.
- Each repetition of the sequence should take 1 to 3 seconds. Repeat as a continuous, controlled, fluid sequence 10 to 12 times.

breathe **Exhale while rounding the shoulders and reaching forward; inhale each time the stretch is released.**

Seated Forward Bend
Trunk extensors

Keep the chin down.

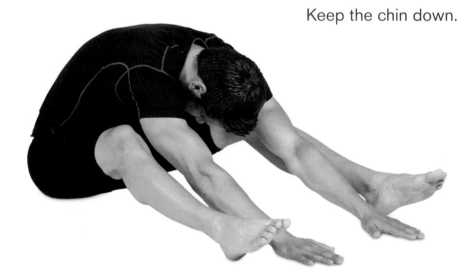

■ Sit on the floor with the knees bent and the legs wide. Drop the chest between the legs toward the floor. Reach forward with the hands on the floor.

■ Hold the stretch for 10 to 30 seconds.

 Exhale deeply while moving into the farthest point of the stretch; then breathe evenly while holding the stretch.

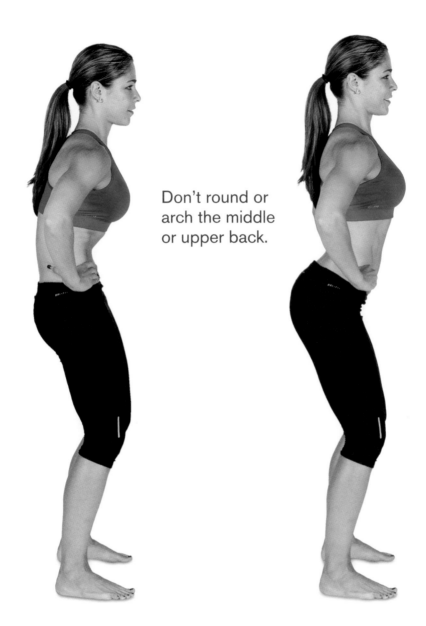

Don't round or
arch the middle
or upper back.

- ▌ Stand with the feet shoulder-width apart.
- ▌ Contract the abs; tuck the tailbone underneath the spine.
- ▌ Release the stretch by contracting the lower back; lift the tailbone out from underneath the spine.
- ▌ Each repetition of the sequence should take 1 to 3 seconds. Repeat as a continuous, controlled, fluid sequence 10 to 12 times.

breathe **Exhale while tucking the tailbone underneath the spine; inhale each time the stretch is released.**

Dynamic Cat
Rhomboids, trunk extensors

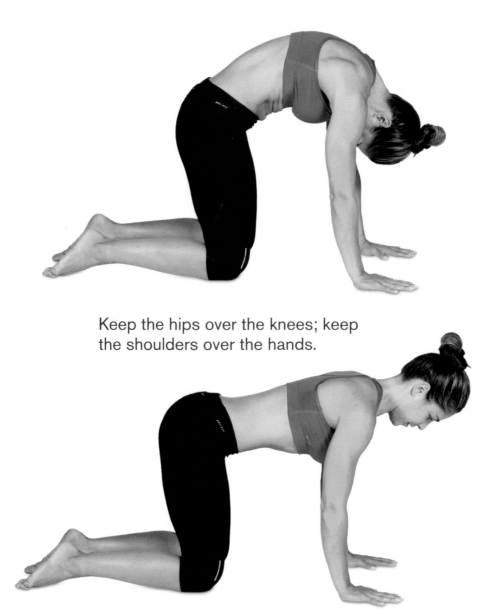

Keep the hips over the knees; keep the shoulders over the hands.

- Kneel on the floor on the hands and the knees.
- Pull in the abdominals to round the spine; tuck the chin into the chest.
- Release the stretch by returning to the start position.
- Each repetition of the sequence should take 1 to 3 seconds. Repeat as a continuous, controlled, fluid sequence 10 to 12 times.

 breathe **Exhale while rounding the spine; inhale each time the stretch is released.**

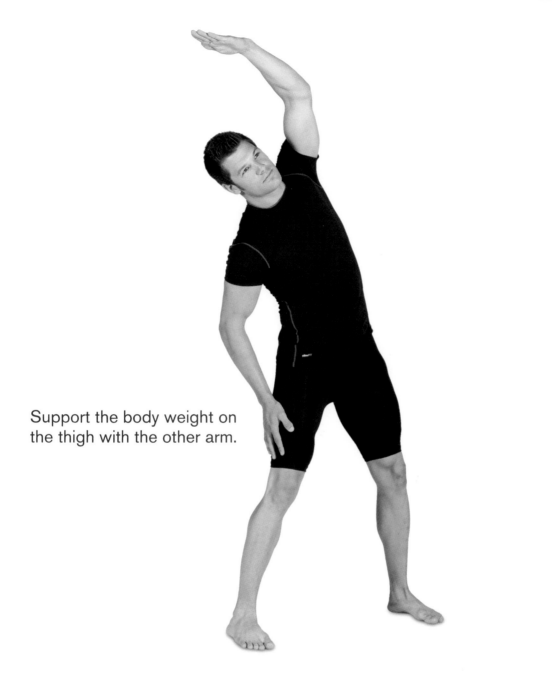

Support the body weight on the thigh with the other arm.

- Stand with the feet apart and the knees slightly bent. Reach with one hand above the head and lean over to the opposite side.
- Hold the stretch for 10 to 30 seconds.
- Repeat on the other side.

breathe **Exhale deeply while moving into the farthest point of the stretch; then breathe evenly while holding the stretch.**

Wall Reach

passive **Latissimus dorsi, lateral trunk flexors**

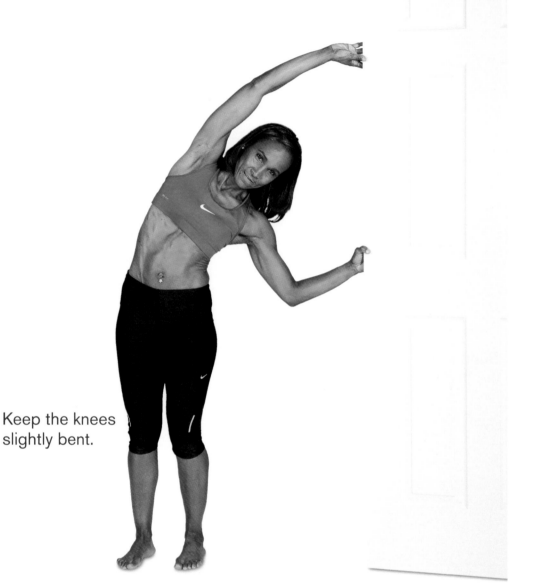

Keep the knees
slightly bent.

▐ Stand with the feet apart. With one side of the body facing a wall or door,
place both hands on the wall by leaning to the side.

▐ Hold the stretch for 10 to 30 seconds.

▐ Repeat on the other side.

breathe **Exhale deeply while moving into the farthest point of the
stretch; then breathe evenly while holding the stretch.**

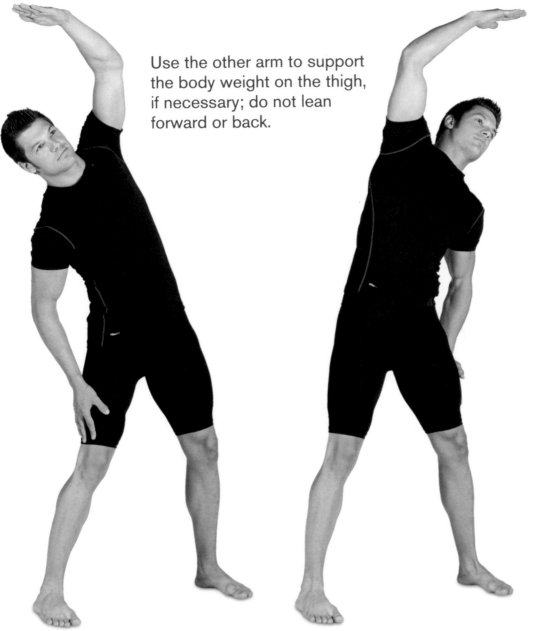

Use the other arm to support the body weight on the thigh, if necessary; do not lean forward or back.

- Stand with the feet apart, the knees slightly bent, and the arms at the sides of the body.
- Reach one hand above the head; lean over to the opposite side.
- Release the stretch by returning to the start position.
- Repeat on the other side.
- Each repetition of the sequence should take 1 to 3 seconds. Repeat as a continuous, controlled, fluid sequence 10 to 12 times.

Exhale while reaching above the head; inhale each time the stretch is released.

Seated Twist

Thoracic-lumbar rotators

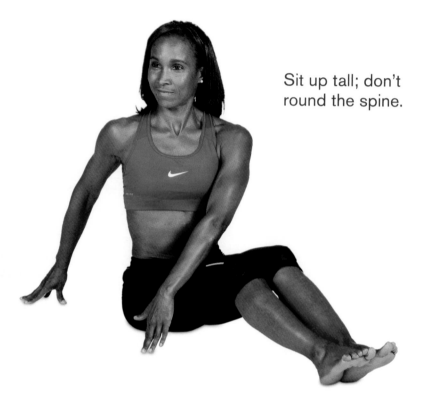

Sit up tall; don't
round the spine.

- Sitting on the floor, extend the legs straight out in front with the knees slightly bent. Place one hand on the floor behind the body and the other across the thigh. Twist the upper body to one side.
- Hold the stretch for 10 to 30 seconds.
- Repeat on the other side.

breathe **Exhale deeply while moving into the farthest point of the stretch; then breathe evenly while holding the stretch.**

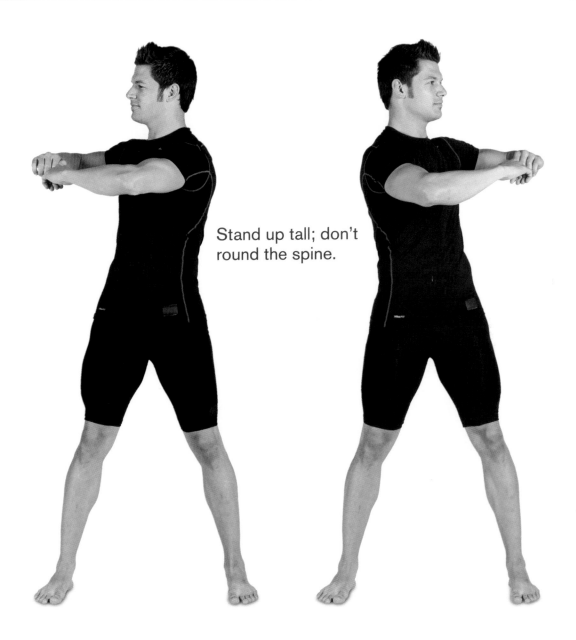

Stand up tall; don't round the spine.

- Stand with the feet shoulder-width apart. Bend the elbows; hold the arms out to the sides.
- Twist the upper body to one side as far as comfortably possible.
- Release the stretch by returning to the start position.
- Repeat on the other side.
- Each repetition of the sequence should take 1 to 3 seconds. Repeat as a continuous, controlled, fluid sequence 10 to 12 times.

 breathe **Exhale while twisting the upper body to the side; inhale each time the stretch is released.**

Double Knee Hug

Trunk extensors, latissimus dorsi, rhomboids, gluteals

Keep the elbows close to the body
and the shoulders relaxed.

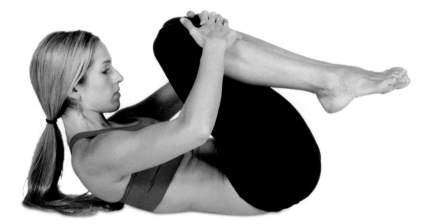

- Lie on the floor face up. Bend the knees and pull the thighs toward the chest while tucking the chin and lifting the shoulders off the floor as high as comfortably possible.

- Hold the stretch for 10 to 30 seconds.

 Exhale deeply while moving into the farthest point of the stretch; then breathe evenly while holding the stretch.

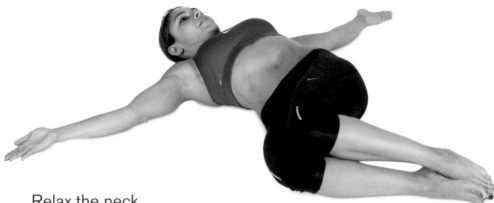

Relax the neck
and the shoulders.

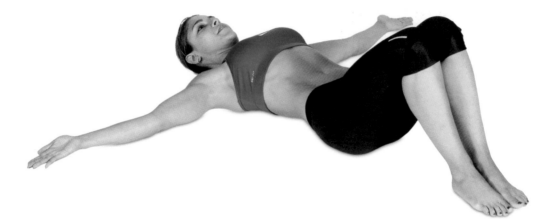

- Lie on the floor face up with the knees bent and the arms extended to the sides of the body at chest height.
- Rotate the hips and the knees to one side of the body as far as comfortably possible.
- Release the stretch by returning to the start position.
- Each repetition of the sequence should take 1 to 3 seconds. Repeat as a continuous, controlled, fluid sequence 10 to 12 times.
- Repeat on the other side.

breathe

Exhale while rotating the hips and the knees; inhale each time the stretch is released.

Side Reach (Ball)

Latissimus dorsi, lateral trunk flexors

Don't lean forward or back. Keep the neck in line with the spine.

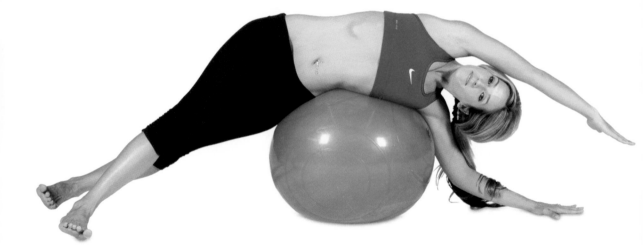

- Place one side of the upper body on the center of a stability ball with the feet on the floor in a split stance. Place the lower arm on the floor for balance and extend the top arm above the head and toward the floor.
- Hold the stretch for 10 to 30 seconds.
- Repeat on the other side.

breathe **Exhale deeply while moving into the farthest point of the stretch; then breathe evenly while holding the stretch.**

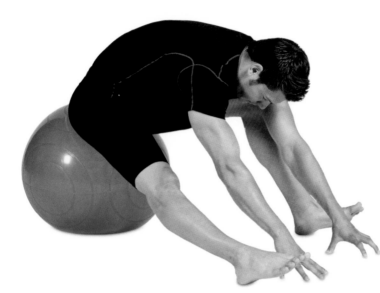

Relax the neck and the shoulders. Keep the chin down.

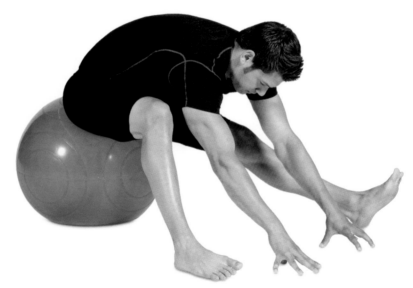

- Sit on the center of a stability ball with the feet flat on the floor and the knees bent. Drop the chest between the legs toward the floor. Reach forward toward the floor.
- Shift the hips to one side by straightening the opposite leg.
- Release the stretch by returning to the start position.
- Repeat on the other side.
- Each repetition of the sequence should take 1 to 3 seconds. Repeat as a continuous, controlled, fluid sequence 10 to 12 times.

breathe **Exhale while shifting the hips to one side; inhale each time the stretch is released.**

Abdominals

Along with the muscles of the lower back, the abdominal muscles help hold us upright throughout the day. These muscles are essential for supporting, protecting, and stabilizing the spine. Performing abdominal stretches helps keep your abdominal muscles flexible and strong, aiding everyday movement and function.

Cobra

passive **Abdominals**

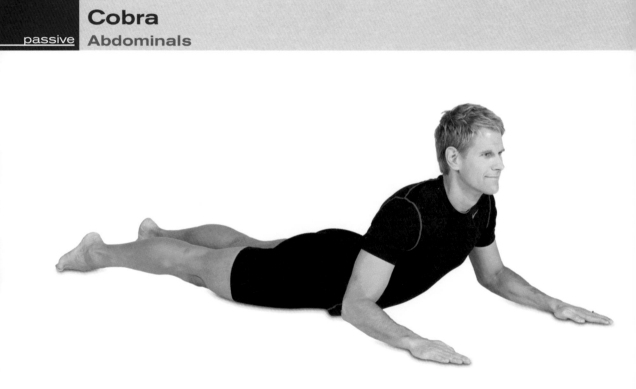

Don't extend beyond the point that's comfortable for the lower back; don't lift the head too far back.

▮ Lie on the floor chest down with the hands near the shoulders. Lift the chest and ribs off the floor as far as comfortably possible by pushing with the hands.

▮ Hold the stretch for 10 to 30 seconds.

breathe **Exhale deeply while moving into the farthest point of the stretch; then breathe evenly while holding the stretch.**

Don't extend beyond the point that's comfortable for the lower back.

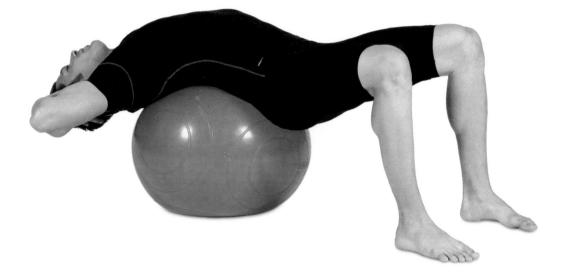

- Place the middle back on the center of a stability ball with the feet out in front and the hands interlaced behind the head. Lower the tailbone, the upper back, and the head around the ball.
- Hold the stretch for 10 to 30 seconds.

 breathe **Exhale deeply while moving into the farthest point of the stretch; then breathe evenly while holding the stretch.**

Don't extend beyond the point that's
comfortable for the lower back.

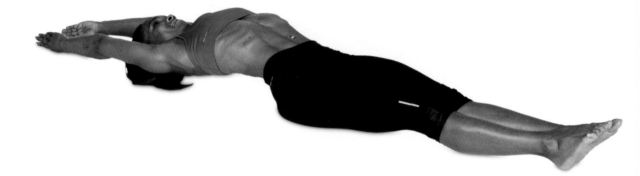

■ Lie on the floor face up with the legs and the arms extended out. Reach as far
away from the center of the body as comfortably possible while gently arching
the lower back and lifting the ribs and the chest toward the ceiling.

■ Hold the stretch for 10 to 30 seconds.

breathe **Exhale deeply while moving into the farthest point of the
stretch; then breathe evenly while holding the stretch.**

Don't extend beyond the point that's comfortable for the lower back; don't lift the head too far back.

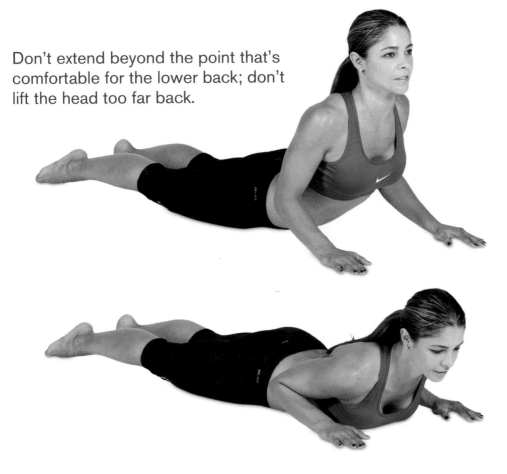

- Lie on the floor face down with the hands in front of the body.
- Lift the chest and the ribs off the floor by contracting the back muscles.
- Release the stretch by returning to the start position.
- Each repetition of the sequence should take 1 to 3 seconds. Repeat as a continuous, controlled, fluid sequence 10 to 12 times.

breathe **Exhale while lifting the chest off the floor; inhale each time the stretch is released.**

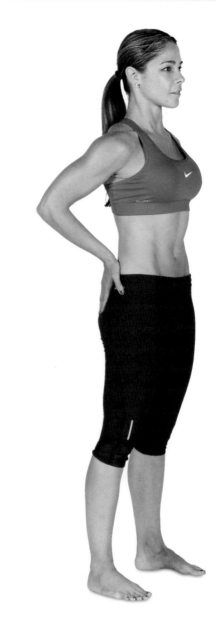

Don't extend
beyond the
point that's
comfortable
for the lower
back; don't
lift the head
too far back.

- ▋ Stand tall with the palms of the hands around the sides of the lower back.
- ▋ Lift the chest and the ribs toward the ceiling by contracting the back muscles and extending the spine.
- ▋ Release the stretch by returning to the start position.
- ▋ Each repetition of the sequence should take 1 to 3 seconds. Repeat as a continuous, controlled, fluid sequence 10 to 12 times.

breathe

Exhale while lifting the chest toward the ceiling; inhale each time the stretch is released.

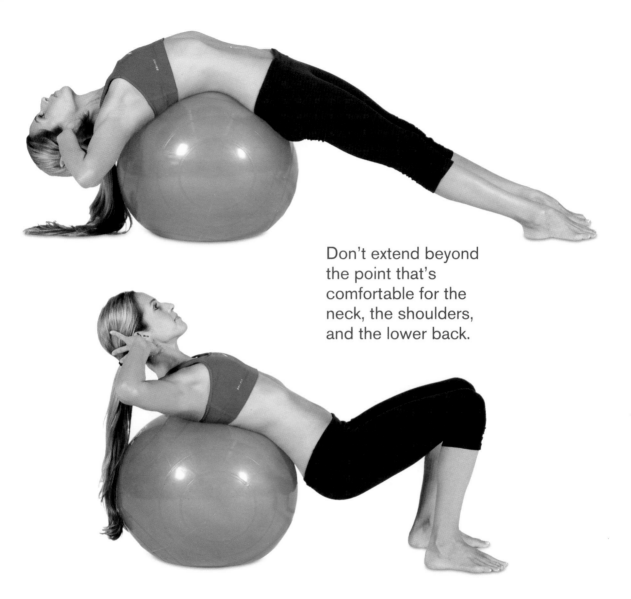

Don't extend beyond the point that's comfortable for the neck, the shoulders, and the lower back.

■ Place the middle back on the front top side of a stability ball with the feet flat on the floor, the knees bent, and the hands behind the head.

■ Roll back over the ball until the legs are almost or completely straight. Lower the tailbone, the upper back, and the head around the ball.

■ Release the stretch by returning to the start position.

■ Each repetition of the sequence should take 1 to 3 seconds. Repeat as a continuous, controlled, fluid sequence 10 to 12 times.

 Exhale while rolling back over the ball; inhale each time the stretch is released.

Ball Cobra
Abdominals

Don't extend beyond the point that's comfortable for the lower back; don't lift the head too far back.

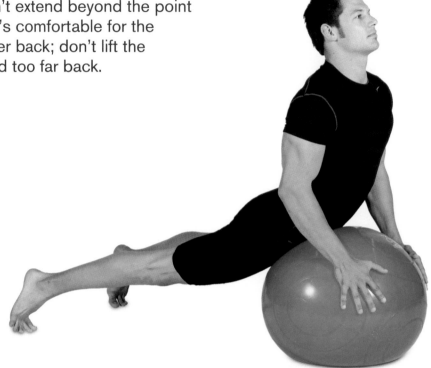

- Lie face down on the center of a stability ball. Place the hands on the front side of the ball, below the shoulders. Raise the chest as high as comfortably possible by pushing against the ball with both hands.
- Hold the stretch for 10 to 30 seconds.

 breathe **Exhale deeply while moving into the farthest point of the stretch; then breathe evenly while holding the stretch.**

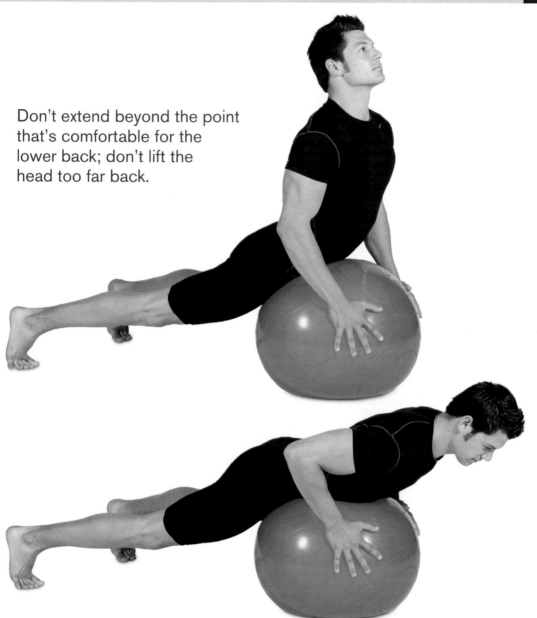

Don't extend beyond the point that's comfortable for the lower back; don't lift the head too far back.

- Lie face down on the center of a stability ball. Place the hands on the front side of the ball, below the shoulders.
- Lift the chest off the ball by contracting the back muscles.
- Release the stretch by returning to the start position.
- Each repetition of the sequence should take 1 to 3 seconds. Repeat as a continuous, controlled, fluid sequence 10 to 12 times.

breathe **Exhale while lifting the chest off the ball; inhale each time the stretch is released.**

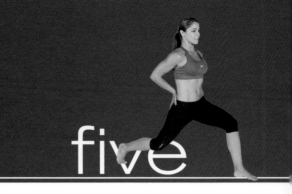

five

Glutes, Hips, and Inner Thighs

This chapter focuses on the muscles that surround, stabilize, and support the pelvis, the gluteals, and the muscles of the hips and inner thighs. These muscles are often the tightest muscles in active people and athletes. Tightness in these muscles can cause aggravation and pain in the lower back and make it uncomfortable to sit for long periods of time. As is true for the quadriceps and hamstrings, imbalanced flexibility in the glutes and hips can lead to problems that travel up the body into the back or down the lower body into the knees. The stretches in this chapter deliver relief and mobility to this important region of the body.

Glutes and Hips

The glutes and hips comprise a great number of muscles that engage every time you sit down, stand up, or climb the stairs. These muscles also work to stabilize the pelvis for many activities, such as those that involve bending over or leaning sideways. Stretching these muscles frequently helps counteract the stress these activities create in this area of the body.

Lying Figure 4
Gluteals, piriformis

Keep the head on the floor.

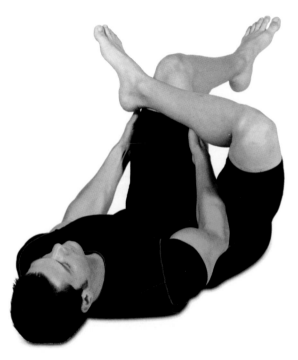

- Lie on the floor face up with the legs bent. Place one foot across the thigh of the opposite leg in the figure-4 position. Reach for the leg on the floor and pull it toward the chest.
- Hold the stretch for 10 to 30 seconds.
- Repeat the stretch with the other leg.

breathe **Exhale deeply while moving into the farthest point of the stretch; then breathe evenly while holding the stretch.**

Use the arms to support the back.

- Sitting on the floor, extend one leg straight out in front; place the foot of the other leg across the thigh in the figure-4 position. Move the chest toward the legs, pivoting at the hips.
- Hold the stretch for 10 to 30 seconds.
- Repeat the stretch with the other leg.

breathe   **Exhale deeply while moving into the farthest point of the stretch; then breathe evenly while holding the stretch.**

Seated Figure 4 on Chair
Gluteals, piriformis

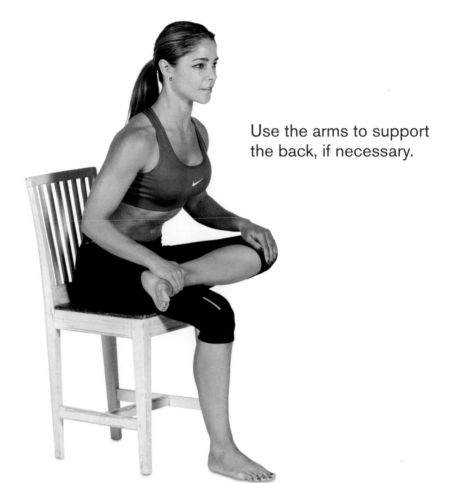

Use the arms to support
the back, if necessary.

■ Sit in a chair with one foot across the thigh of the opposite leg in the figure-4
position. Move the chest toward the legs, pivoting at the hips.

■ Hold the stretch for 10 to 30 seconds.

■ Repeat the stretch with the other leg.

breathe **Exhale deeply while moving into the farthest point of the
stretch; then breathe evenly while holding the stretch.**

Relax the head and the neck.

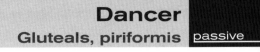

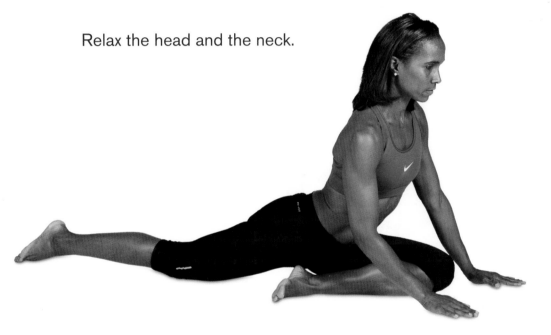

▌ Lie on the floor face down. Raise the upper body off the floor, resting on the hands. Bend one knee and bring it underneath the opposite leg.

▌ Hold the stretch for 10 to 30 seconds.

▌ Repeat the stretch with the other leg.

 Exhale deeply while moving into the farthest point of the stretch; then breathe evenly while holding the stretch.

Standing Figure 4
Gluteals, piriformis

Hold onto something stable for balance, if necessary. Keep the head up. Don't round the spine.

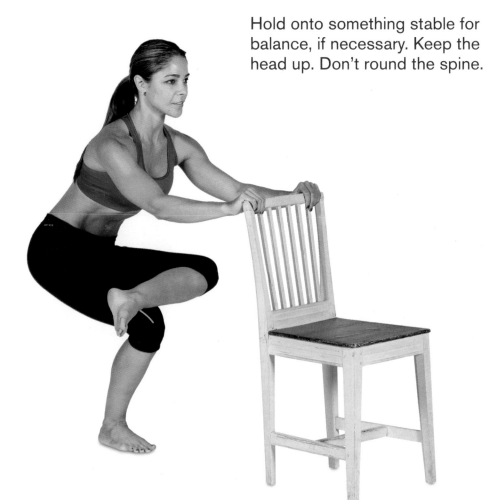

- Stand with the feet slightly apart. Place one foot across the thigh of the opposite leg in the figure-4 position. Squat down.
- Hold the stretch for 10 to 30 seconds.
- Repeat the stretch with the other leg.

breathe

Exhale deeply while moving into the farthest point of the stretch; then breathe evenly while holding the stretch.

Hip Push
Gluteals, piriformis passive

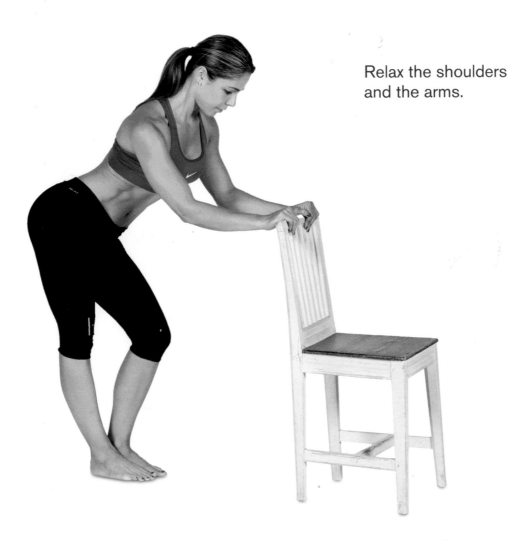

Relax the shoulders
and the arms.

- Stand with the feet together, holding onto a chair. Bend forward slightly at the waist. Bend one leg and straighten the other, pushing the straight-leg hip outward.
- Hold the stretch for 10 to 30 seconds.
- Repeat the stretch with the other leg.

 Exhale deeply while moving into the farthest point of the stretch; then breathe evenly while holding the stretch.

Dynamic Knee Hug
Gluteals

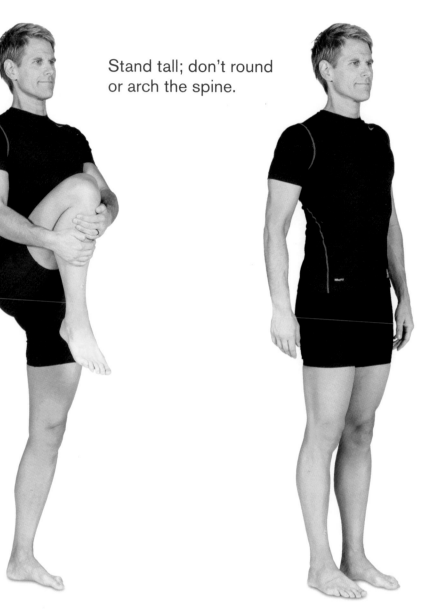

Stand tall; don't round or arch the spine.

- Stand with the feet together. Bring one knee forward and up toward the chest.
- Place the hands around the shin and pull the knee into the chest.
- Release the stretch by putting the foot on the floor.
- Each repetition of the sequence should take 1 to 3 seconds. Repeat as a continuous, controlled, fluid sequence 10 to 12 times.
- Repeat the stretch with the other leg.

 breathe **Exhale while pulling the knee into the chest; inhale each time the stretch is released.**

Dynamic Lying Figure-4 Circle

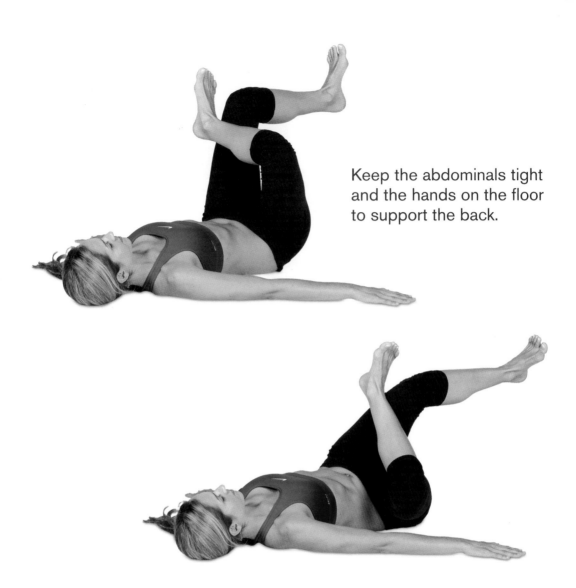

Keep the abdominals tight and the hands on the floor to support the back.

▮ Lie on the floor on the back with knees bent. Place one foot across the thigh of the opposite leg in the figure-4 position. Lift the other foot off the floor and rotate the leg in a circular motion.

▮ Each repetition of the sequence should take 1 to 3 seconds. Repeat as a continuous, controlled, fluid sequence 10 to 12 times.

▮ Repeat the sequence with the other leg.

breathe **Breathe evenly while performing the sequence.**

Dynamic Hip Push
Gluteals, piriformis

Relax the shoulders
and the arms.

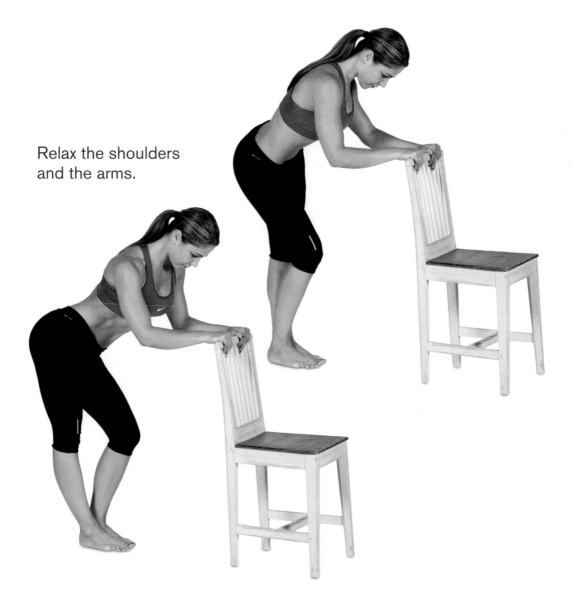

- Standing with the feet together, bend the elbows and hold onto a chair with the hands. Bend forward slightly at the waist.
- Bend one leg and straighten the other, pushing the straight-leg hip outward.
- Release the stretch by returning to the start position.
- Each repetition of the sequence should take 1 to 3 seconds. Repeat as a continuous, controlled, fluid sequence 10 to 12 times.
- Switch the legs and repeat the sequence.

breathe **Exhale while pushing the hip outward; inhale each time the stretch is released.**

Keep the abdominals tight
and the hands on the floor
to support the back.

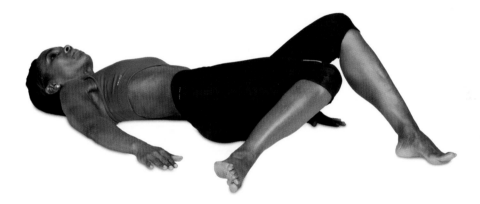

- Lie on the back face up with the knees bent, soles of the feet on the floor, and the knees touching. Lift one leg slightly, and drop the other knee inward toward the floor.

- Hold the stretch for 10 to 30 seconds.

- Repeat the stretch with the other leg.

breathe **Exhale deeply while moving into the farthest point of the stretch; then breathe evenly while holding the stretch.**

Dynamic Lying Crossover
Hip rotators (internal)

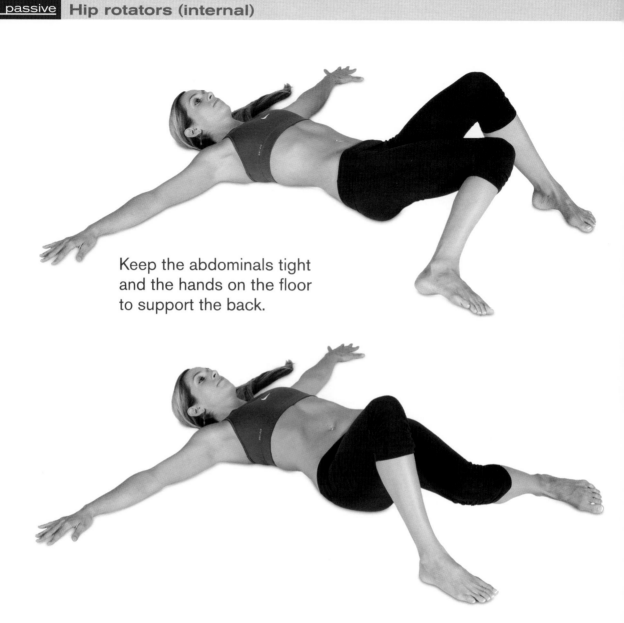

Keep the abdominals tight
and the hands on the floor
to support the back.

- Lie on the back face up with the knees bent, soles of the feet on the floor, and the knees touching.
- Lift one leg slightly; drop the other knee inward toward the floor.
- Release the stretch by returning to the start position.
- Each repetition of the sequence should take 1 to 3 seconds. Repeat as a continuous, controlled, fluid sequence 10 to 12 times.
- Repeat the stretch with the other leg.

breathe **Exhale while dropping the knee inward; inhale each time the stretch is released.**

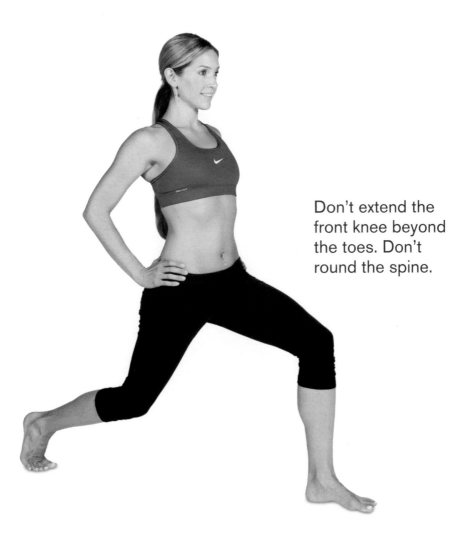

Don't extend the
front knee beyond
the toes. Don't
round the spine.

■ Stand tall with the legs in a lunge position. Lower the back knee toward the
floor and tilt the hips toward the ceiling.

■ Hold the stretch for 10 to 30 seconds.

■ Repeat the stretch with the other leg.

breathe **Exhale deeply while moving into the farthest point of the
stretch; then breathe evenly while holding the stretch.**

Kneeling Runner's Lunge
Hip flexors

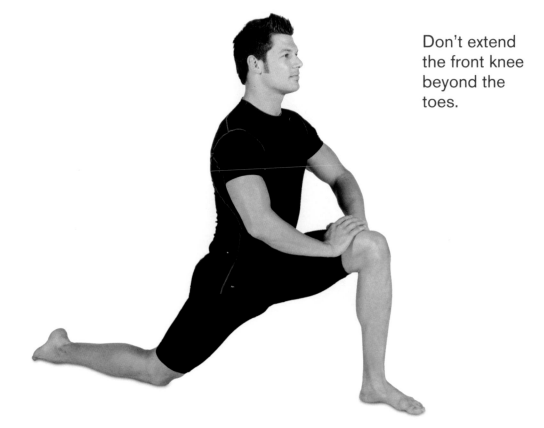

Don't extend the front knee beyond the toes.

- Kneel on one leg. Step out with the front foot and gently press the hips forward. Place the hands on the front thigh for support, if necessary.
- Hold the stretch for 10 to 30 seconds.
- Repeat the stretch with the other leg.

breathe **Exhale deeply while moving into the farthest point of the stretch; then breathe evenly while holding the stretch.**

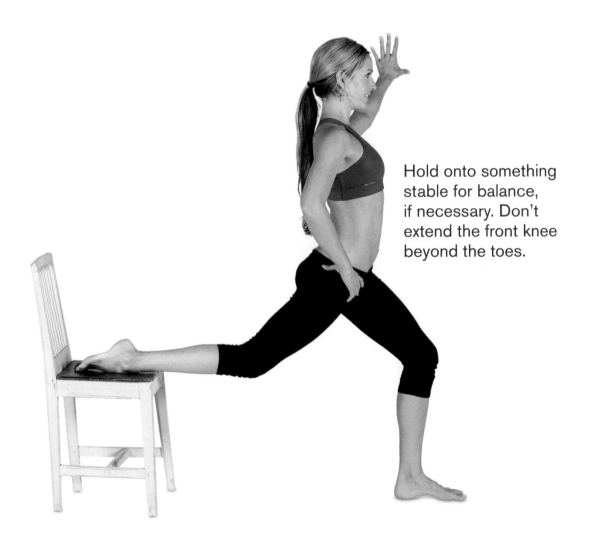

Hold onto something stable for balance, if necessary. Don't extend the front knee beyond the toes.

- Stand tall and place one foot behind on a chair or bench. Bend the front leg and push the hips forward.
- Hold the stretch for 10 to 30 seconds.
- Repeat the stretch with the other leg.

 Exhale deeply while moving into the farthest point of the stretch; then breathe evenly while holding the stretch.

Dynamic Lying Leg Lift
Hip flexors

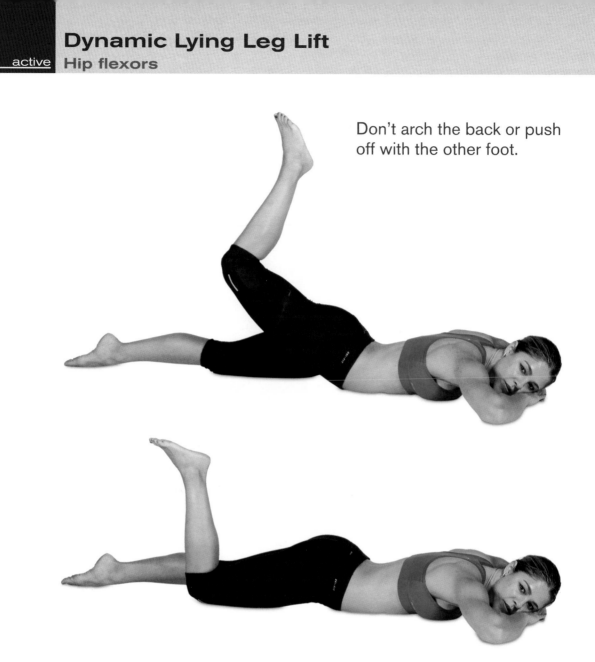

Don't arch the back or push off with the other foot.

- Lie on the floor face down. Turn the head to one side. Bend one knee until the sole of the foot faces the ceiling.
- Lift the front of the thigh off the floor as high as comfortably possible.
- Release the stretch by lowering the thigh back to the floor.
- Each repetition of the sequence should take 1 to 3 seconds. Repeat as a continuous, controlled, fluid sequence 10 to 12 times.
- Repeat the stretch with the other leg.

breathe **Exhale while lifting the front of the thigh off the floor; inhale each time the stretch is released.**

Don't lean forward while extending the leg behind.
Hold onto something stable for balance, if necessary.

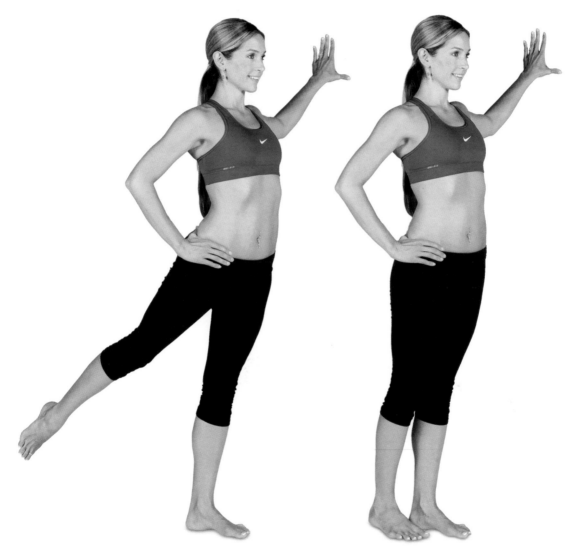

- Stand tall.
- Straighten one leg and extend it behind the body as far as comfortably possible.
- Release the stretch by returning to the start position.
- Each repetition of the sequence should take 1 to 3 seconds. Repeat as a continuous, controlled, fluid sequence 10 to 12 times.
- Repeat the stretch with the other leg.

 breathe **Exhale while extending the leg behind the body; inhale each time the stretch is released.**

Inner Thighs

The muscles of the inner thigh tend to be tight and weak for many people because they don't get used as aggressively or as often as other muscle groups. The risks associated with tight or weak inner thigh muscles are generally small in typical daily activities but prove significant if you're involved in activities such as soccer, in-line skating, or horseback riding. Strong, flexible inner thigh muscles help minimize injuries from falls and groin strains.

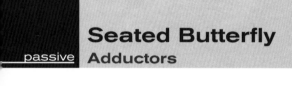

Seated Butterfly

passive **Adductors**

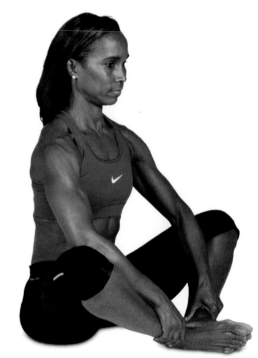

Don't round
the spine.

▌ Sit on the floor with the soles of the feet together. Place the forearms or the elbows on the inner thighs; bring the chest slightly toward the legs. Pivot from the hips and push the thighs toward the floor.

▌ Hold the stretch for 10 to 30 seconds.

 breathe **Exhale deeply while moving into the farthest point of the stretch; then breathe evenly while holding the stretch.**

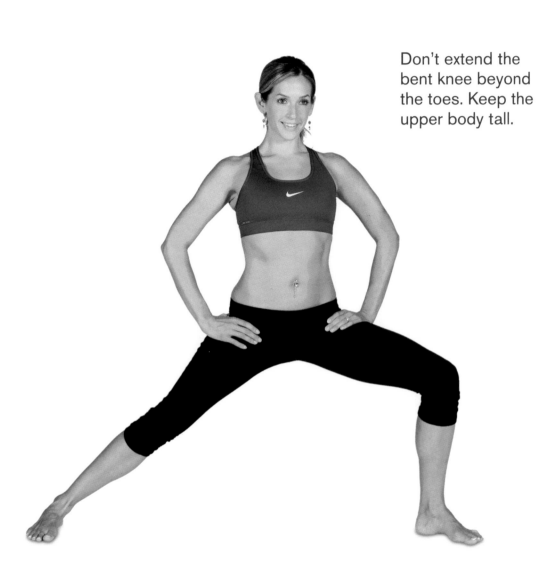

Don't extend the bent knee beyond the toes. Keep the upper body tall.

- Stand with the feet wide apart. Bend one knee and lunge to the same side, keeping the other leg straight.
- Hold the stretch for 10 to 30 seconds.
- Repeat the stretch with the other leg.

breathe **Exhale deeply while moving into the farthest point of the stretch; then breathe evenly while holding the stretch.**

Sumo Squat
Adductors

Don't drop
the hips
below the
knees.

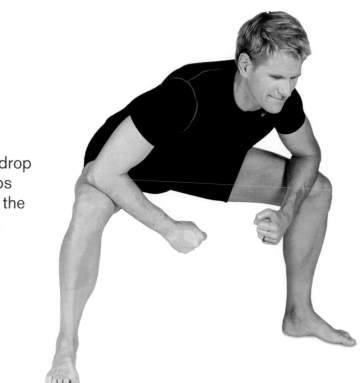

■ Stand with the feet wide apart and the toes turned out. Sit down into a low
squat position. Lean the upper body forward; use the forearms to press against
the inside of the thighs.

■ Hold the stretch for 10 to 30 seconds.

 breathe **Exhale deeply while moving into the farthest point of the
stretch; then breathe evenly while holding the stretch.**

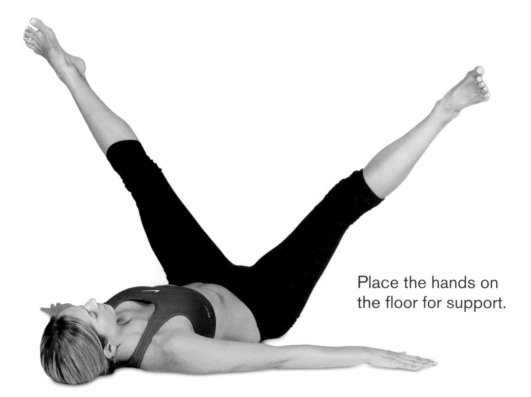

Place the hands on
the floor for support.

❚ Lie on the floor face up with the legs in the air and the knees slightly bent.
Slowly open the legs and lower them toward the floor.

❚ Hold the stretch for 10 to 30 seconds.

breathe

**Exhale deeply while moving into the farthest point of the
stretch; then breathe evenly while holding the stretch.**

Seated Straddle
Adductors

Support the back
with the arms.

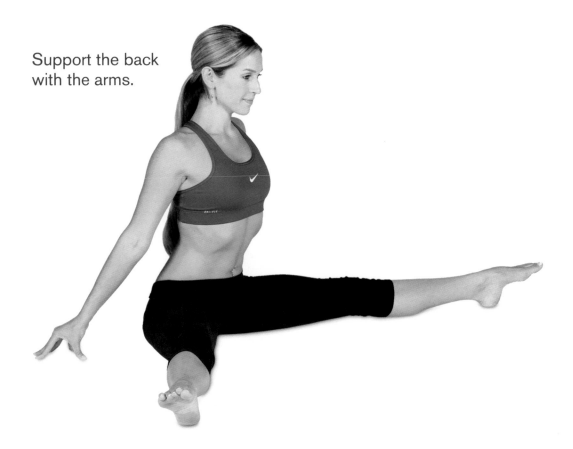

▋ Extend the legs straight out in front with the knees slightly bent. Open the legs
as wide as comfortably possible.

▋ Hold the stretch for 10 to 30 seconds.

 breathe **Exhale deeply while moving into the farthest point of the
stretch; then breathe evenly while holding the stretch.**

Don't arch the back.

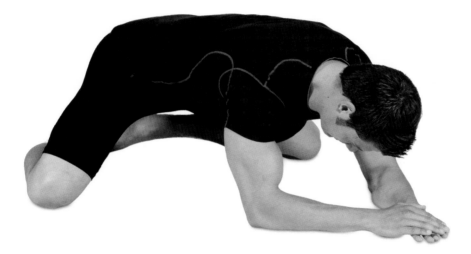

- Kneeling on the floor, keep the feet together and open the knees as wide as comfortably possible. Rest the upper body on the elbows.
- Hold the stretch for 10 to 30 seconds.

 breathe **Exhale deeply while moving into the farthest point of the stretch; then breathe evenly while holding the stretch.**

Dynamic Seated Butterfly
Adductors

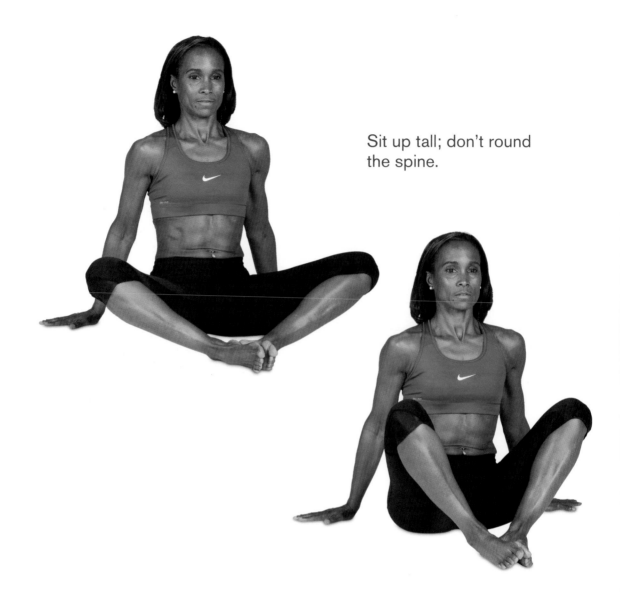

Sit up tall; don't round the spine.

- Sit on the floor and bring the soles of the feet together.
- Pull the knees to the floor by contracting the outside of the thighs.
- Release the stretch by returning to the start position.
- Each repetition of the sequence should take 1 to 3 seconds. Repeat as a continuous, controlled, fluid sequence 10 to 12 times.

breathe **Exhale while pulling the knees toward the floor; inhale each time the stretch is released.**

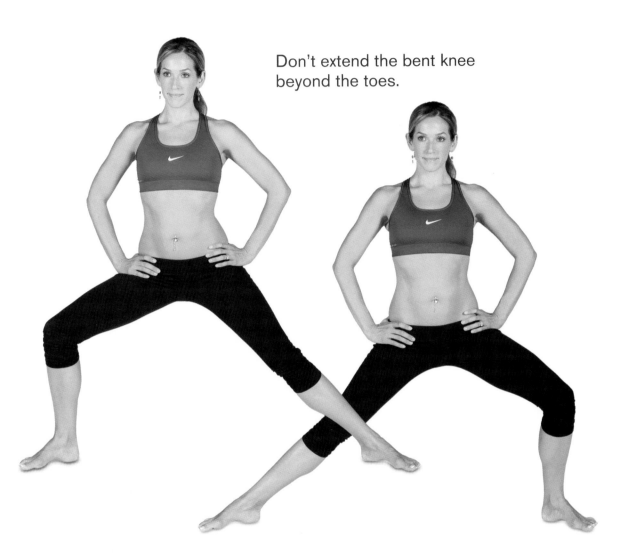

Don't extend the bent knee beyond the toes.

- Stand with the feet wide apart.
- Bend one knee and lunge to the same side. Contract the gluteals on the opposite side and keep that leg straight.
- Release the stretch by returning to the start position.
- Each repetition of the sequence should take 1 to 3 seconds. Repeat as a continuous, controlled, fluid sequence 10 to 12 times.
- Repeat on the other side.

breathe **Exhale while lunging to the side; inhale each time the stretch is released.**

Dynamic Seated Straddle

Adductors

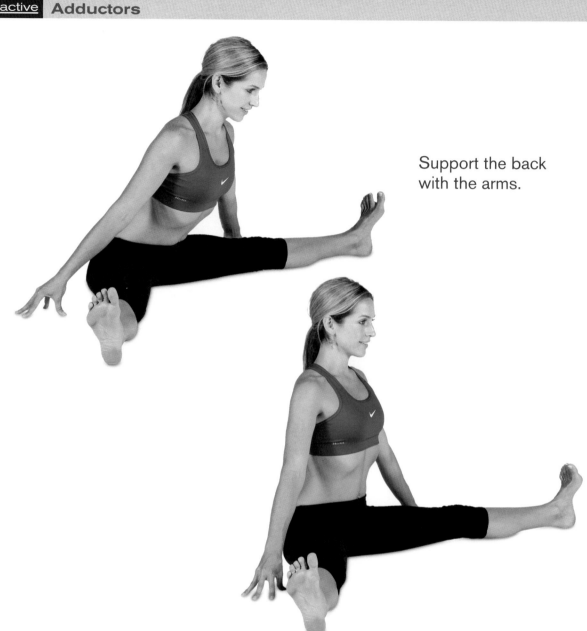

Support the back
with the arms.

- Extend the legs straight in front with the knees slightly bent. Open the legs as wide as possible.
- Contract the gluteals. Lean forward, pivoting at the hips.
- Release the stretch by returning to the start position.
- Each repetition of the sequence should take 1 to 3 seconds. Repeat as a continuous, controlled, fluid sequence 10 to 12 times.

breathe **Exhale while leaning forward; inhale each time the stretch is released.**

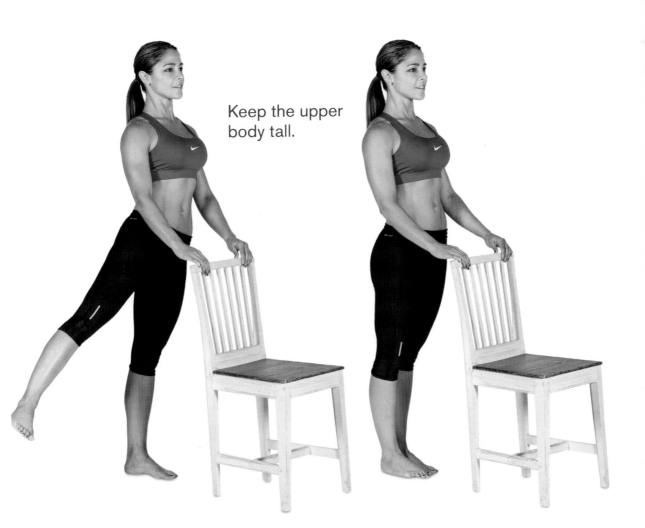

Keep the upper body tall.

- Standing with the feet together, touch the back of a chair with the palms of the hands.
- Raise one leg out to the side as high as comfortably possible.
- Release the stretch by returning to the start position.
- Each repetition of the sequence should take 1 to 3 seconds. Repeat as a continuous, controlled, fluid sequence 10 to 12 times.
- Repeat the stretch with the other leg.

breathe **Exhale while raising the leg out to the side; inhale each time the stretch is released.**

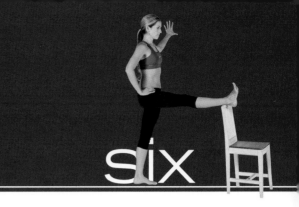

six

Quadriceps and Hamstrings

This chapter focuses on the large muscles that cover the front and back of the upper leg. These muscles are among the strongest, most powerful in the body and are frequently sore and tight from running, cycling, jumping, and other activities. Imbalanced flexibility in these muscles can lead to problems that travel up the body into the back or down the lower body into the knees.

Quadriceps

The quadriceps are a group of four very strong muscles that make up the front of the thigh. We use them in nearly every sport and in everyday movements, such as standing up, sitting down, and walking. Although the quadriceps are not overly tight for most people, they are often fatigued or sore. Stretching these muscles feels good and improves mobility around the knee joint.

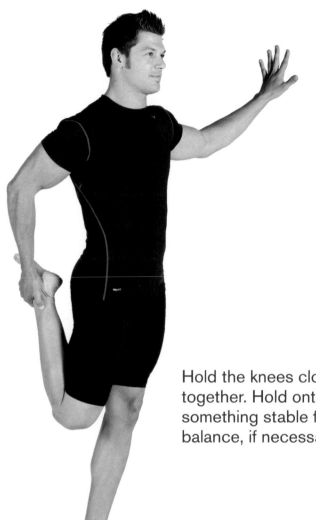

Hold the knees close together. Hold onto something stable for balance, if necessary.

- Stand with the feet together. Bend one knee and hold the ankle with the same-side hand; pull the heel toward the gluteals.
- Hold the stretch for 10 to 30 seconds.
- Repeat on the other leg.

breathe **Exhale deeply while moving into the farthest point of the stretch; then breathe evenly while holding the stretch.**

Side-Lying Knee Bend
Quadriceps

Hold the knees close together.

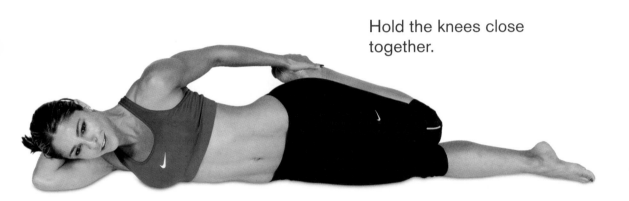

- Lie on one side, resting the head on the lower arm. Bend the top knee and hold the ankle with the same-side hand; pull the heel toward the gluteals.
- Hold the stretch for 10 to 30 seconds.
- Lie on the other side and repeat the stretch with the other leg.

breathe **Exhale deeply while moving into the farthest point of the stretch; then breathe evenly while holding the stretch.**

Anchored Knee Bend

Quadriceps

Hold onto something stable for balance, if necessary.

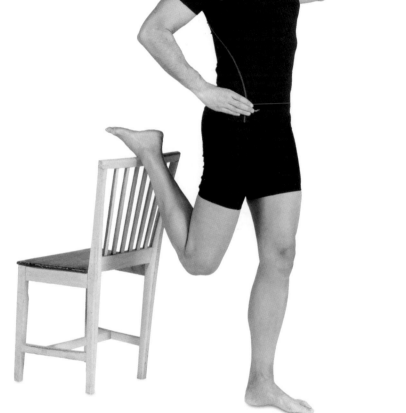

- Stand with the feet together facing away from the back of a chair. Bend one knee and place the top of the foot on the back of the chair.
- Hold the stretch for 10 to 30 seconds.
- Repeat the stretch with the other leg.

 Exhale deeply while moving into the farthest point of the stretch; then breathe evenly while holding the stretch.

112

Dynamic Side-Lying Knee Bend

Quadriceps active

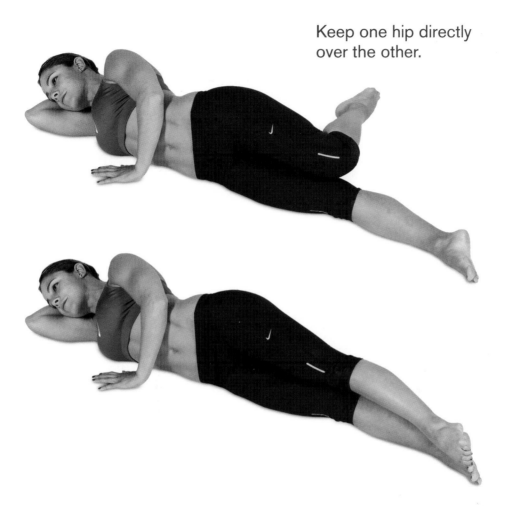

Keep one hip directly over the other.

- Lie on one side, resting the head on the lower arm.
- Bend the top leg at the knee, bringing the heel toward the gluteals.
- Release the stretch by returning the leg to the start position.
- Each repetition of the sequence should take 1 to 3 seconds. Repeat as a continuous, controlled, fluid sequence 10 to 12 times.
- Lie on the other side and repeat the stretch with the other leg.

breathe **Exhale while bringing the heel toward the gluteals; inhale each time the stretch is released.**

Dynamic Lying Knee Bend
Quadriceps

Keep the upper body relaxed.

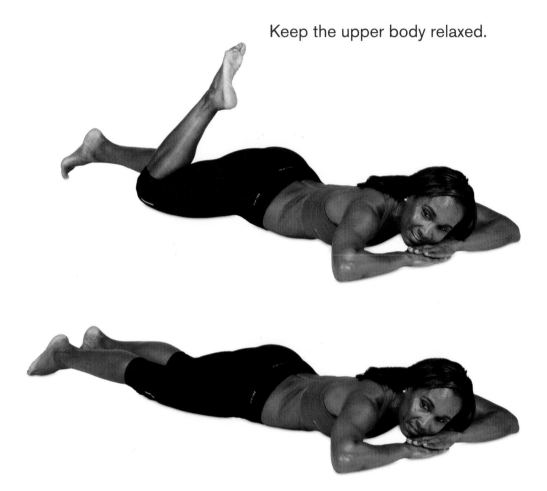

- Lie face down with the legs extended and the head turned to one side, resting on the back of the hands.
- Bend the knee of one leg and move the heel toward the gluteals.
- Release the stretch by returning the leg to the start position.
- Each repetition of the sequence should take 1 to 3 seconds. Repeat as a continuous, controlled, fluid sequence 10 to 12 times.
- Repeat the stretch with the other leg.

breathe **Exhale while bringing the heel toward the gluteals; inhale each time the stretch is released.**

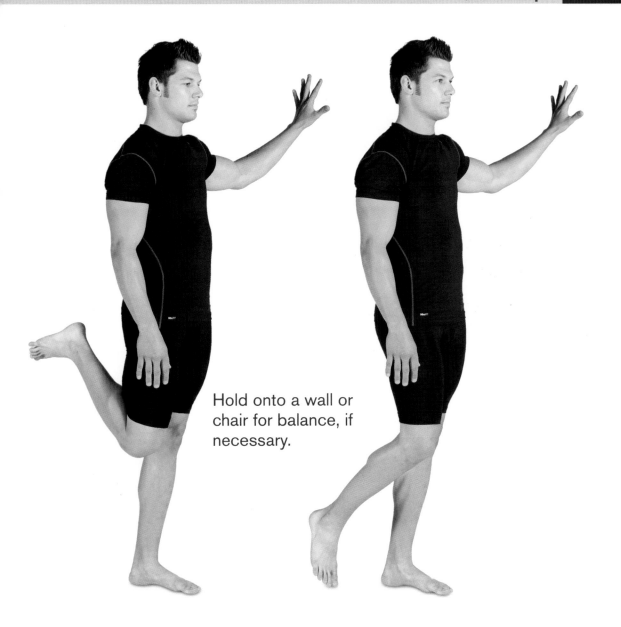

Hold onto a wall or chair for balance, if necessary.

- Stand with the feet together.
- Raise the heel of one foot toward the gluteals.
- Release the stretch by returning the leg to the start position.
- Each repetition of the sequence should take 1 to 3 seconds. Repeat as a continuous, controlled, fluid sequence 10 to 12 times.
- Repeat the stretch with the other leg.

breathe **Exhale while bringing the heel toward the gluteals; inhale each time the stretch is released.**

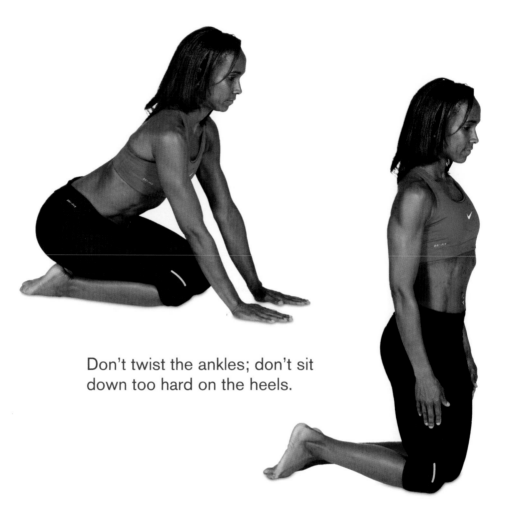

Don't twist the ankles; don't sit down too hard on the heels.

- Kneel on the floor with the toes down, the heels up, and the body upright.
- Sit back on the heels as far as comfortably possible; place the hands on the floor in front of the body.
- Release the stretch by returning to the start position.
- Each repetition of the sequence should take 1 to 3 seconds. Repeat as a continuous, controlled, fluid sequence 10 to 12 times.

breathe **Exhale while sitting back on the heels; inhale each time the stretch is released.**

Don't twist the ankles; don't sit down too hard on the heels.

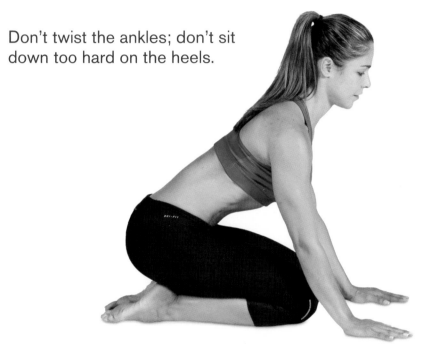

- Kneel on the floor with the toes down, the heels up, and the body upright. Sit back on the heels as far as comfortably possible and place the hands on the floor in front of the body.
- Hold the stretch for 10 to 30 seconds.

breathe **Exhale deeply while moving into the farthest point of the stretch; breathe evenly while holding the stretch.**

Hamstrings

The hamstring muscles make up the back of the thigh. They work in partnership with the quadriceps to bend and straighten the knee and extend the hip. Many people have tight hamstrings from sitting so much during the day (the seated position shortens the hamstrings), and the hamstrings can become sore fairly easily from movements such as lunging, squatting, sprinting, and leaping. Strong, flexible hamstrings improve mobility around the hip and knee joints and make nearly all activities easier and more comfortable.

Lying Leg Raise
passive **Hamstrings**

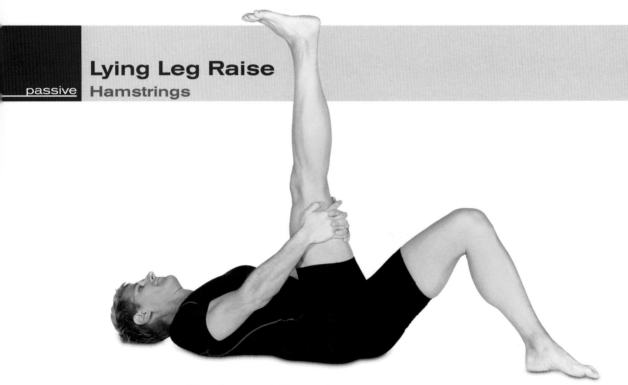

Don't round the spine.

▮ Lie on the floor face up with the legs slightly bent. Lift one leg, keeping the knee straight. Place the hand (or a strap) around the thigh and move the leg closer to the head.

▮ Hold the stretch for 10 to 30 seconds.

▮ Repeat the stretch with the other leg.

 Exhale deeply while moving into the farthest point of the stretch; then breathe evenly while holding the stretch.

Don't lift the head
too far back.

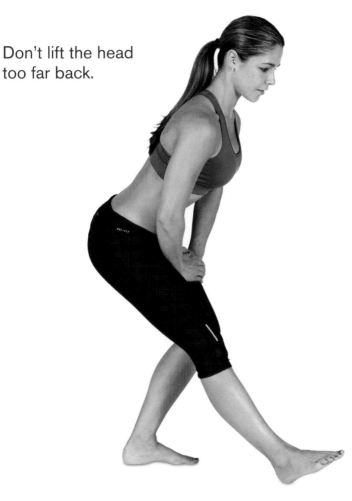

- Stand with one foot forward and one foot back. Straighten the front leg and bend the back knee. Lean forward, pivoting at the hips, and place the hands on the thigh of the bent knee.
- Hold the stretch for 10 to 30 seconds.
- Repeat the stretch with the other leg.

 breathe **Exhale deeply while moving into the farthest point of the stretch; then breathe evenly while holding the stretch.**

Don't round the spine. Keep the knees straight, but don't lock them.

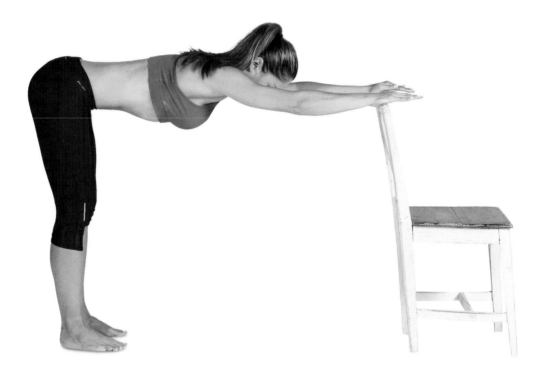

■ Stand with the feet together facing a wall or chair. Lean forward, pivoting at the hips, keeping the knees straight. Use the wall or chair to support the weight of the upper body.

■ Hold the stretch for 10 to 30 seconds.

breathe **Exhale deeply while moving into the farthest point of the stretch; then breathe evenly while holding the stretch.**

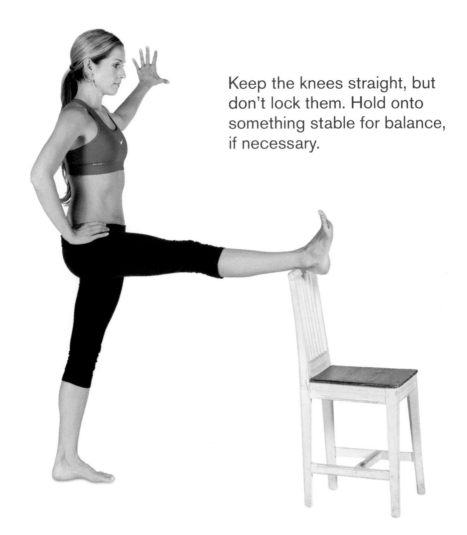

Keep the knees straight, but don't lock them. Hold onto something stable for balance, if necessary.

▮ Stand with the feet together facing the back of a chair. Raise one leg and rest it on top of the back of the chair. Stand tall and straighten the knee.

▮ Hold the stretch for 10 to 30 seconds.

▮ Repeat the stretch with the other leg.

breathe **Exhale deeply while moving into the farthest point of the stretch; then breathe evenly while holding the stretch.**

Dynamic Knee Kick

Hamstrings

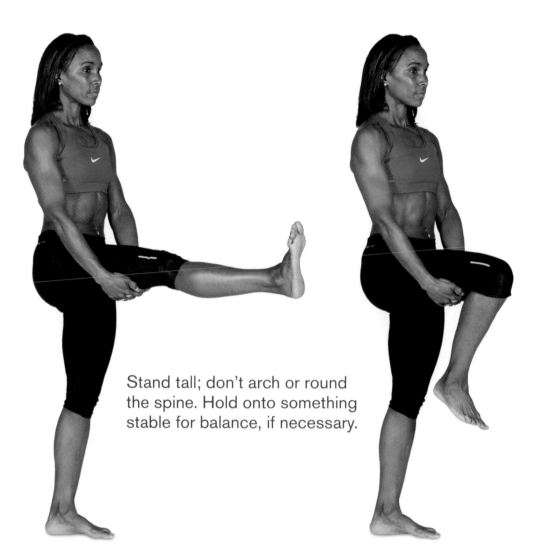

Stand tall; don't arch or round the spine. Hold onto something stable for balance, if necessary.

- Stand tall and hold one leg up with the hands at hip height, keeping the knee bent.
- Straighten the knee as far as comfortably possible.
- Release the stretch by returning to the start position.
- Each repetition of the sequence should take 1 to 3 seconds. Repeat as a continuous, controlled, fluid sequence 10 to 12 times.
- Repeat the stretch with the other leg.

breathe **Exhale while straightening the knee; inhale each time the stretch is released.**

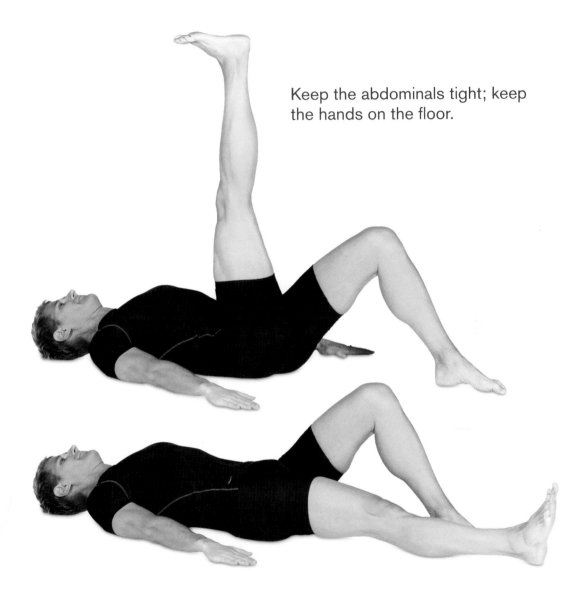

Keep the abdominals tight; keep the hands on the floor.

- Lie on the floor face up with one knee bent and one leg straight.
- Lift the straight leg toward the chest as far as comfortably possible.
- Release the stretch by returning to the start position.
- Each repetition of the sequence should take 1 to 3 seconds. Repeat as a continuous, controlled, fluid sequence 10 to 12 times.
- Repeat the sequence with the other leg.

Exhale while lifting the leg toward the chest; inhale each time the stretch is released.

Dynamic Lying Knee Kick
Hamstrings

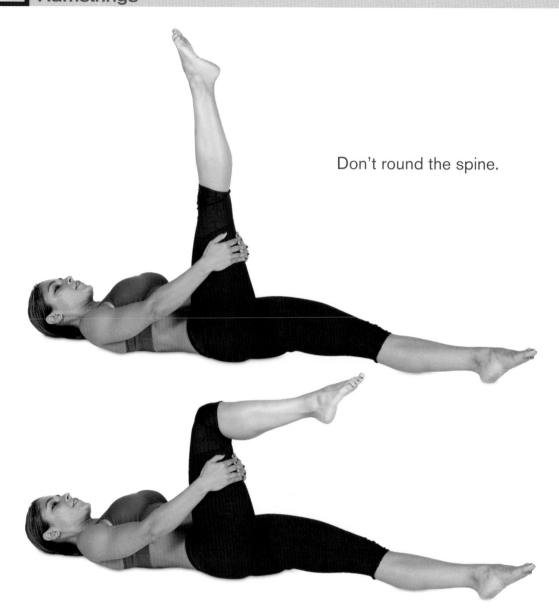

Don't round the spine.

- Lie on the floor face up holding one leg up with the hands and the knee bent. Straighten the other leg.
- Straighten the knee as much as comfortably possible.
- Release the stretch by returning to the start position.
- Each repetition of the sequence should take 1 to 3 seconds. Repeat as a continuous, controlled, fluid sequence 10 to 12 times.
- Repeat the stretch with the other leg.

breathe

Exhale while straightening the knee; inhale each time the stretch is released.

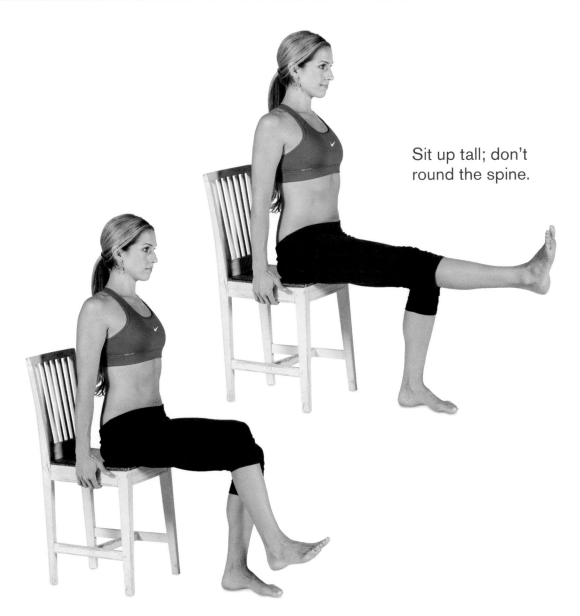

Sit up tall; don't round the spine.

- Sit up straight in a chair.
- Raise one foot slightly off the floor and straighten the knee as much as comfortably possible.
- Release the stretch by returning to the start position.
- Each repetition of the sequence should take 1 to 3 seconds. Repeat as a continuous, controlled, fluid sequence 10 to 12 times.
- Repeat the stretch with the other leg.

breathe **Exhale while straightening the knee; inhale each time the stretch is released.**

125

Dynamic Rolling Ball Knee Kick
Hamstrings

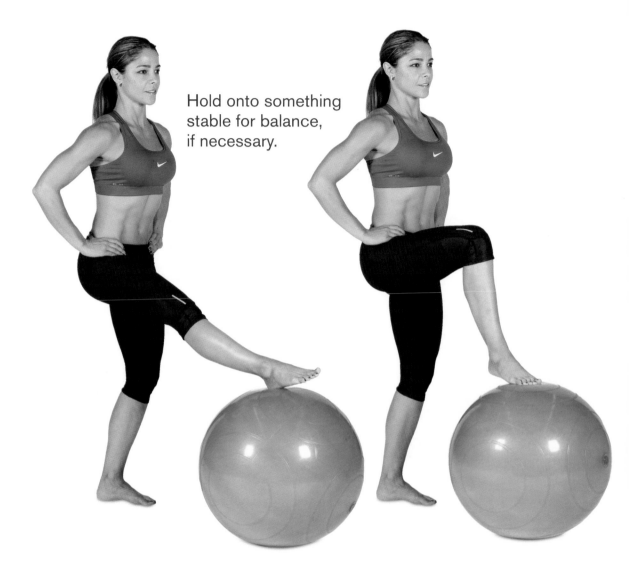

Hold onto something stable for balance, if necessary.

- Stand tall behind a stability ball with one knee bent and the bottom of the foot on the center of the ball.
- Roll the ball away from the body while straightening the knee and hinging at the hip.
- Release the stretch by returning to the start position.
- Each repetition of the sequence should take 1 to 3 seconds. Repeat as a continuous, controlled, fluid sequence 10 to 12 times.
- Repeat the stretch with the other leg.

 breathe **Exhale while rolling the ball away from the body; inhale each time the stretch is released.**

Don't round the spine. Keep the knees straight, but don't lock them. Use the arms to support the back, if necessary.

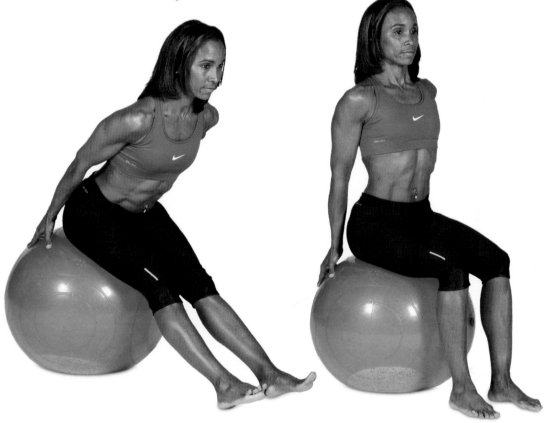

■ Sit tall on the center of a stability ball with the knees bent, the heels on the floor in front of the knees, and the toes up.

■ Roll the ball backward while straightening the knee and hinging at the hips.

■ Release the stretch by returning to the start position.

■ Each repetition of the sequence should take 1 to 3 seconds. Repeat as a continuous, controlled, fluid sequence 10 to 12 times.

breathe **Exhale while rolling the ball backward; inhale each time the stretch is released.**

Hip Hinge (Ball)
Hamstrings

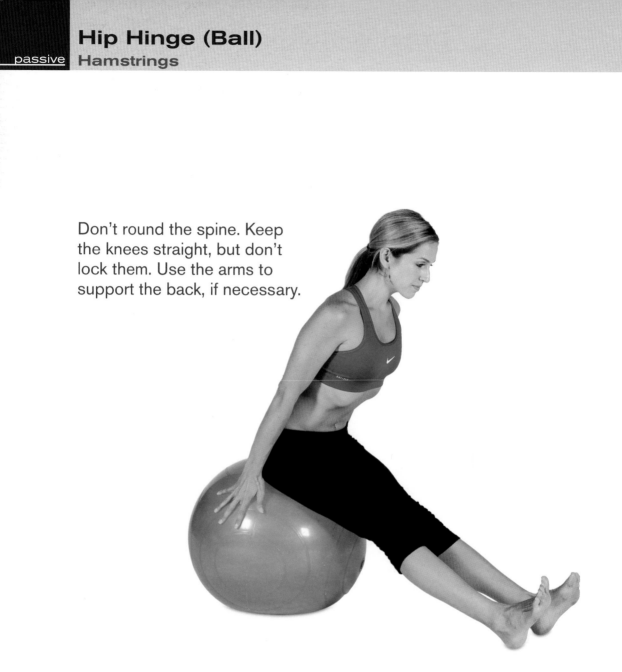

Don't round the spine. Keep the knees straight, but don't lock them. Use the arms to support the back, if necessary.

- Sit tall on the center of a stability ball with the legs extended straight in front of the body, the heels on the floor, and the toes up. Move the chest toward the legs, pivoting at the hips.
- Hold the stretch for 10 to 30 seconds.

 breathe **Exhale deeply while moving into the farthest point of the stretch; breathe evenly while holding the stretch.**

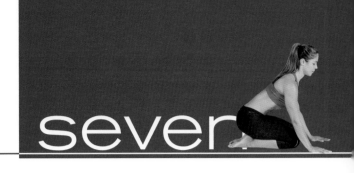

seven

Calves, Shins, and Feet

This chapter focuses on the muscles of the lower legs and feet. Most of the impact forces on our body (that come from the activities we do and sports we play) begin in these muscle groups. These muscle groups act almost like shock absorbers, taking on a great deal of mechanical stress for the rest of the body. As a result, these areas tend to require extra attention, and yet they are often neglected. All of us have had sore feet, calves, or shin pain at some time in our lives. These stretches reduce the incidence and severity of this type of stress. The stretches feel good and allow you to stay on your feet for longer periods of time.

Calves

The calf is the generic name for the two muscles in the back of your lower leg—the gastrocnemius (upper calf) and the soleus (lower calf). The calves are used for pointing the toes and lifting the heels off the ground and are also used explosively in any jumping activity, such as basketball or jumping rope. Women who wear high heels often have inflexible calves because the elevated heel causes the calf to be shortened for long periods of time. These stretches provide mobility around the ankle joint and keep your calves from getting too tight.

Heel Drop

<u>passive</u> **Gastrocnemius**

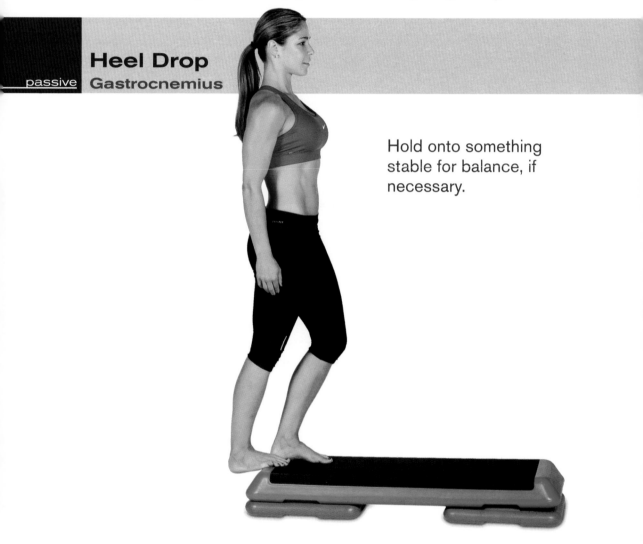

Hold onto something stable for balance, if necessary.

- ▌ Place the ball of the foot on the edge of a step or curb. Push the heel down, keeping the knee straight. Place the other foot slightly in front.
- ▌ Hold the stretch for 10 to 30 seconds.
- ▌ Repeat the stretch with the other foot.

 Exhale deeply while moving into the farthest point of the stretch; then breathe evenly while holding the stretch.

Don't arch the back.

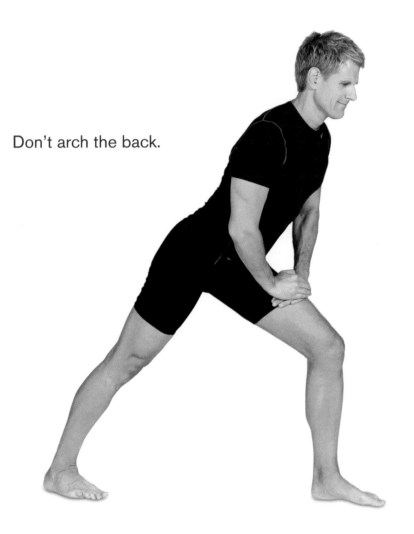

- Stand with one foot forward and one foot back, the legs hip-width apart, the feet facing forward. Bend the front knee and place the hands on the front thigh.
- Hold the stretch for 10 to 30 seconds.
- Repeat the stretch with the other leg.

 Exhale deeply while moving into the farthest point of the stretch; then breathe evenly while holding the stretch.

Toe Up
Gastrocnemius

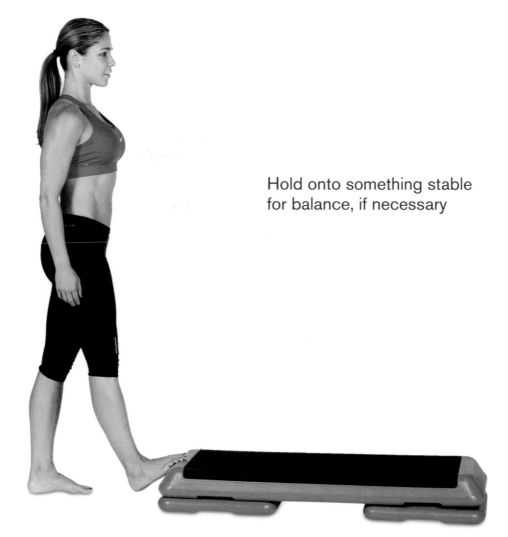

Hold onto something stable
for balance, if necessary

- Stand with the ball of one foot on a curb or step and the other foot flat on the floor behind. Push the hips forward, keeping the knee straight.
- Hold the stretch for 10 to 30 seconds.
- Repeat the stretch with the other foot.

 Exhale deeply while moving into the farthest point of the stretch; then breathe evenly while holding the stretch.

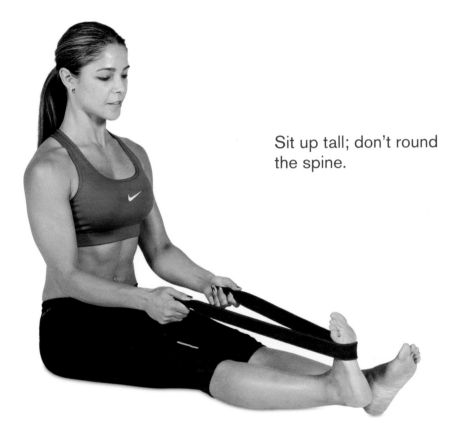

Sit up tall; don't round the spine.

- Sit on the floor, extending the legs straight out in front. Place the stretch strap around the ball of one foot. Use the strap to pull the foot closer to the body.
- Hold the stretch for 10 to 30 seconds.
- Repeat the stretch with the other leg.

 Exhale deeply while moving into the farthest point of the stretch; then breathe evenly while holding the stretch.

Dynamic Seated Flex and Point

Gastrocnemius

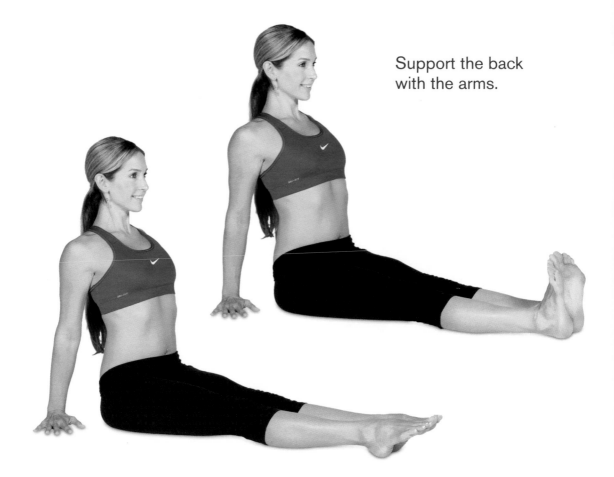

Support the back
with the arms.

- Sit on the floor, extending the legs straight out in front with the knees slightly bent and the toes pointed.
- Flex the feet toward the body.
- Release the stretch by returning to the start position.
- Each repetition of the sequence should take 1 to 3 seconds. Repeat as a continuous, controlled, fluid sequence 10 to 12 times.

 Exhale while flexing the feet toward the body; inhale each time the stretch is released.

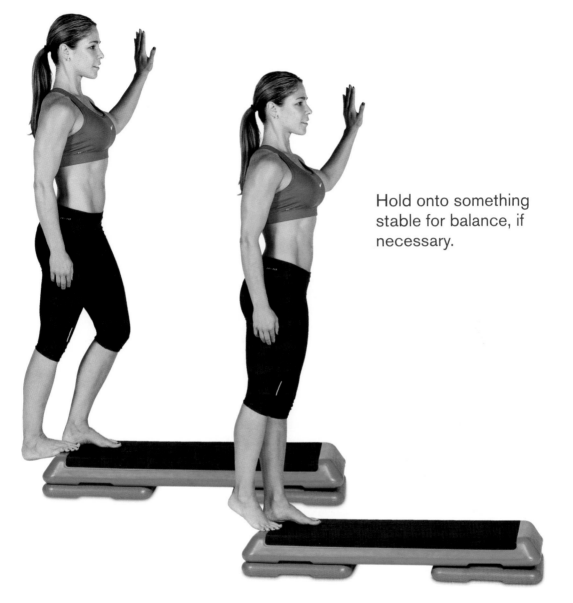

Hold onto something stable for balance, if necessary.

- Place the ball of one foot on the edge of a step or curb. Place the other foot slightly in front.
- Lower the heel, keeping the knee straight.
- Release the stretch by returning to the start position.
- Each repetition of the sequence should take 1 to 3 seconds. Repeat as a continuous, controlled, fluid sequence 10 to 12 times.
- Repeat the sequence with the other leg.

breathe **Exhale while lowering the heel; inhale each time the stretch is released.**

Don't sit down too hard
on the heel. Use the
arms for balance.

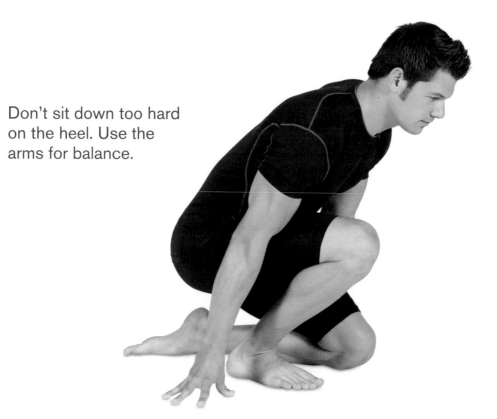

- Kneel down on one knee and sit back on the heel. Place the opposite foot next to the knee, keeping the heel on the floor.
- Hold the stretch for 10 to 30 seconds.
- Repeat the stretch with the other leg.

breathe **Exhale deeply while moving into the farthest point of the stretch; then breathe evenly while holding the stretch.**

Bent-Knee Heel Drop

Achilles tendon, soleus passive

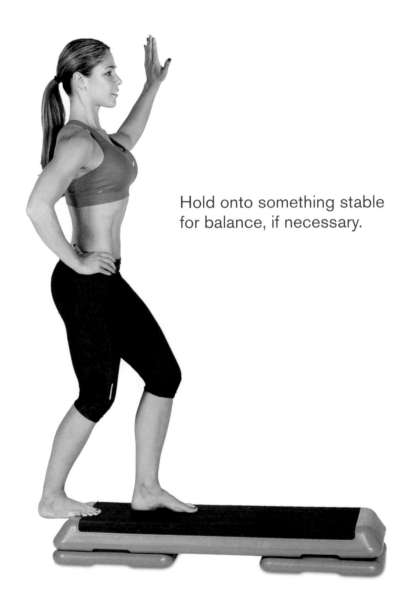

Hold onto something stable for balance, if necessary.

- Place the ball of one foot on the edge of a step or curb. Push the heel down, keeping the knee bent. Place the other foot in front.
- Hold the stretch for 10 to 30 seconds.
- Repeat the stretch with the other foot.

 Exhale deeply while moving into the farthest point of the stretch; then breathe evenly while holding the stretch.

Bent-Knee Heel Press
Achilles tendon, soleus

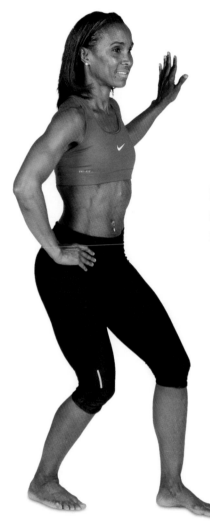

Hold onto something stable for balance, if necessary.

- Stand with one foot forward and one foot back, hip-width apart and the feet facing forward. Bend both knees, putting weight on the back heel.
- Hold the stretch for 10 to 30 seconds.
- Repeat the stretch with the other leg.

 breathe **Exhale deeply while moving into the farthest point of the stretch; then breathe evenly while holding the stretch.**

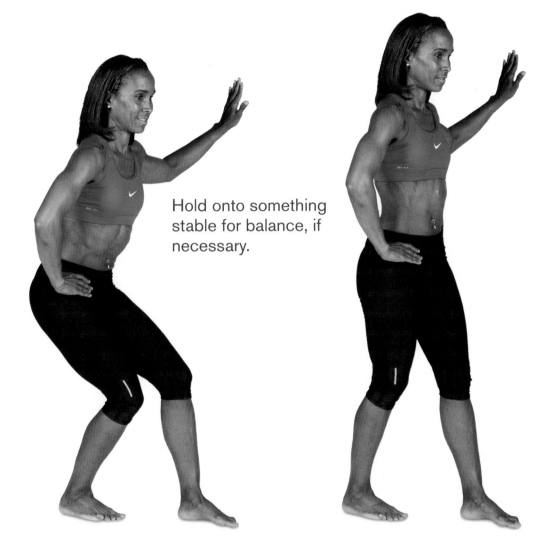

Hold onto something stable for balance, if necessary.

▮ Stand with one foot forward and one foot back, hip-width apart and feet facing forward.

▮ Bend both knees, putting weight on the back heel.

▮ Release the stretch by returning to the start position.

▮ Each repetition of the sequence should take 1 to 3 seconds. Repeat as a continuous, controlled, fluid sequence 10 to 12 times.

▮ Repeat the stretch with the other leg.

breathe **Exhale while bending the knees; inhale each time the stretch is released.**

Dynamic Seated Bent-Knee Flex and Point
Achilles tendon, soleus

Sit up tall; don't round the spine.

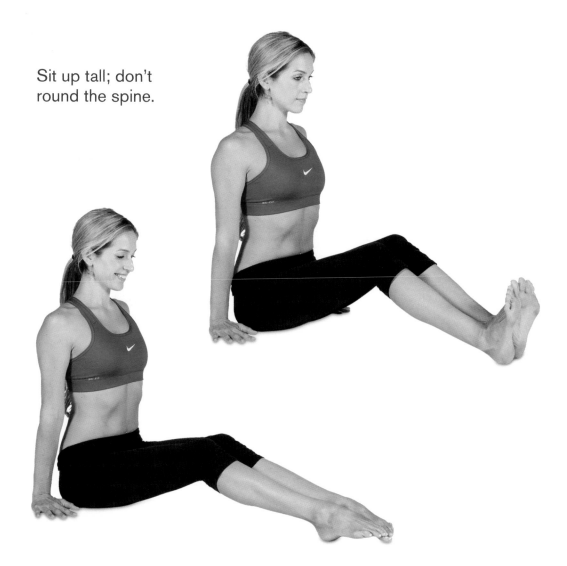

- Sit on the floor, extending the legs straight out in front with the knees bent and the toes pointed.
- Flex the feet toward the body as far as comfortably possible, keeping the knees bent.
- Release the stretch by returning to the start position.
- Each repetition of the sequence should take 1 to 3 seconds. Repeat as a continuous, controlled, fluid sequence 10 to 12 times.

breathe   **Exhale while flexing the foot toward the body; inhale each time the stretch is released.**

Shins

The muscles of the shin work in partnership with the calves to flex and extend the ankle. The shin muscle is often overlooked in daily stretches, but flexible shins help in activities that use the calves. If the shin muscles are flexible, the toes can point farther and the calves can contract with more force, which helps with many sports and everyday activities (e.g., exploding upward for a dunk, reaching up into a high cupboard).

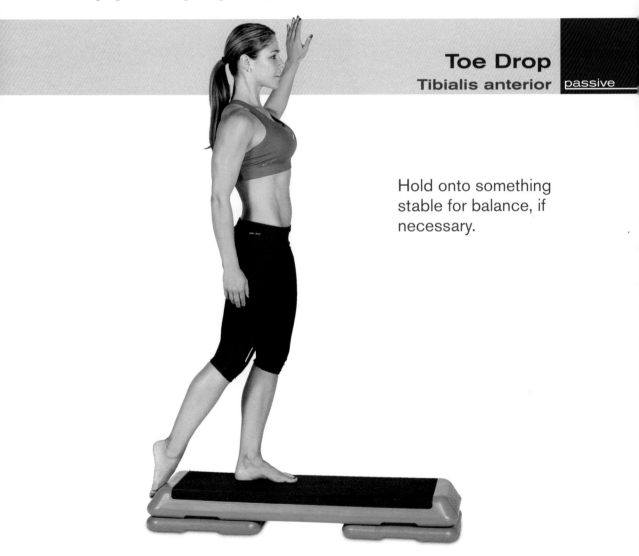

Toe Drop
Tibialis anterior passive

Hold onto something stable for balance, if necessary.

▐ Place the top of one foot against the edge of a step or curb. Place the other foot in front. Press the back leg forward while pointing the toes.

▐ Hold the stretch for 10 to 30 seconds.

▐ Repeat the stretch with the other foot.

breathe

Exhale deeply while moving into the farthest point of the stretch; then breathe evenly while holding the stretch.

Seated Foot Pull
Tibialis anterior

Sit up tall; don't
round the spine.

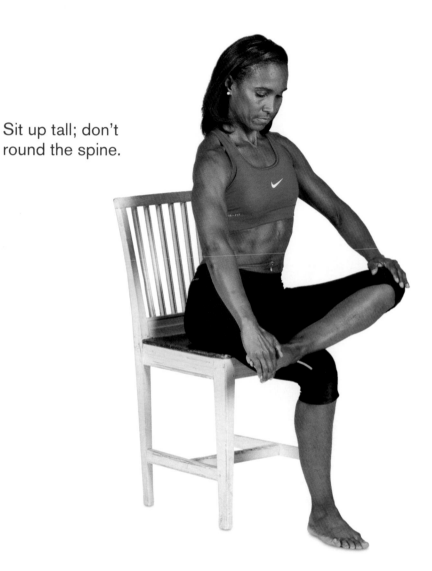

- Sit in a chair and rest one ankle just above the opposite knee. Pull the ball of the foot toward the body without twisting the ankle.
- Hold the stretch for 10 to 30 seconds.
- Repeat the stretch with the other foot.

Exhale deeply while moving into the farthest point of the stretch; then breathe evenly while holding the stretch.

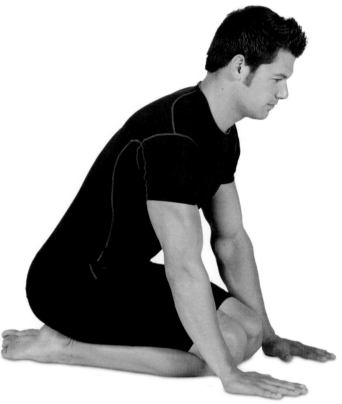

Don't twist the ankles. Don't sit
down too hard on the heels.

- Kneeling on the floor, point the toes and sit back directly on the heels.
- Use the arms to support the upper body.
- Hold the stretch for 10 to 30 seconds.

breathe **Exhale deeply while moving into the farthest point of the
stretch; then breathe evenly while holding the stretch.**

Dynamic Seated Half-Circle
Tibialis anterior

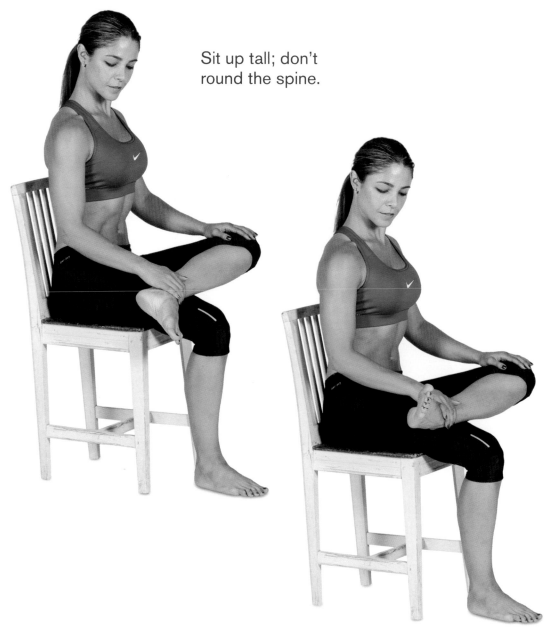

Sit up tall; don't
round the spine.

- Sit in a chair, resting one ankle just above the opposite knee.
- Point the toes.
- Draw the shape of the lower half of a circle with the foot.
- Each repetition of the sequence should take 1 to 3 seconds. Repeat as a continuous, controlled, fluid sequence 10 to 12 times.
- Repeat the sequence with the other foot.

breathe **Breathe evenly while performing the sequence.**

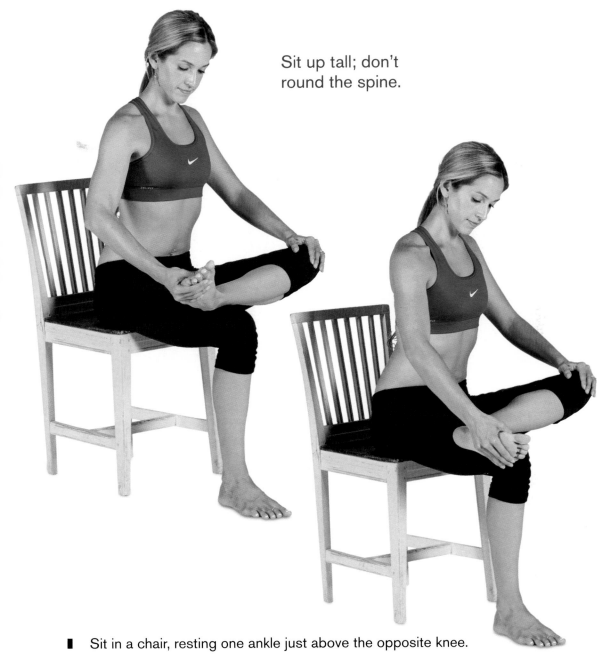

Sit up tall; don't round the spine.

- Sit in a chair, resting one ankle just above the opposite knee.
- Use a hand to move the sole of the foot inward.
- Use a hand to move the sole of the foot outward.
- Each repetition of the sequence should take 1 to 3 seconds. Repeat as a continuous, controlled, fluid sequence 10 to 12 times.
- Repeat the sequence with the other foot.

breathe **Breathe evenly while performing the sequence.**

Dynamic Seated Ankle Roll

active **Ankle rotators**

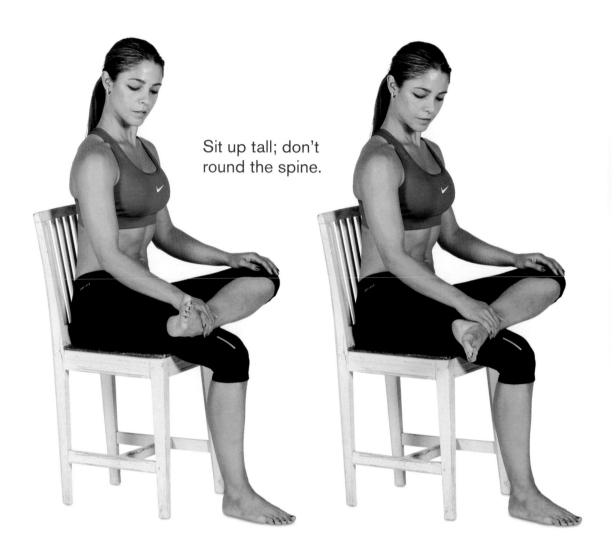

Sit up tall; don't round the spine.

∎ Sit in a chair, resting one ankle just above the opposite knee.

∎ Point the toes.

∎ Draw the shape of a large circle with the foot.

∎ Each repetition of the sequence should take 1 to 3 seconds. Repeat as a continuous, controlled, fluid sequence 10 to 12 times.

∎ Repeat the sequence with the other foot.

breathe **Breathe evenly while performing the sequence.**

Feet

Stretches for the feet feel good and release much of the tension that builds up in these smaller muscle groups. Because these muscles support your body every time you take a step, it is important to perform these simple stretches whenever possible. These stretches are particularly useful if you experience soreness during or after walking, running, or jumping.

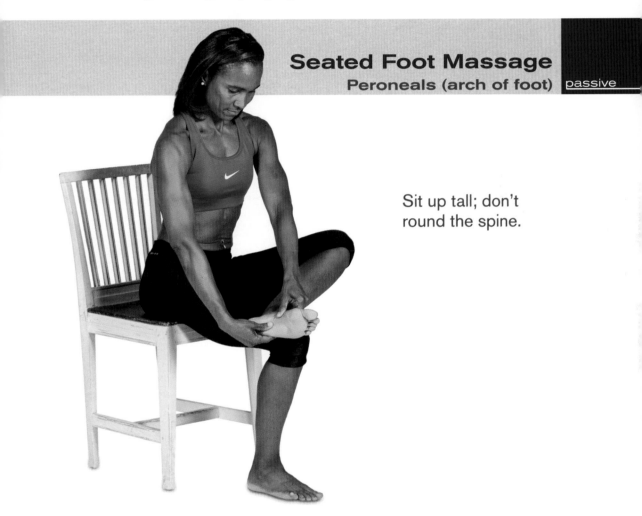

Seated Foot Massage
Peroneals (arch of foot)   passive

Sit up tall; don't round the spine.

- Sit in a chair, resting one ankle just above the opposite knee.
- Gently massage the arch of the foot with the hands. Gradually work deeper into the muscle under the arch.
- Repeat the massage on the other foot.

breathe   **Breathe evenly while performing the sequence.**

Dynamic Seated Toe Flex and Point
Peroneals (arch of foot)

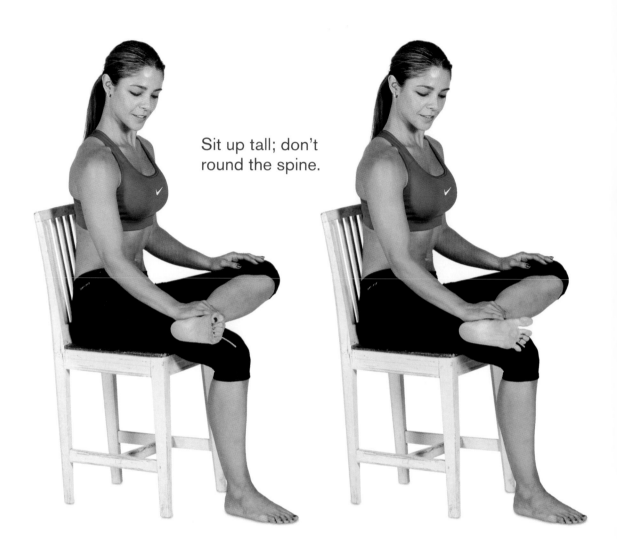

Sit up tall; don't round the spine.

- Sit in a chair, resting one ankle just above the opposite knee.
- Flex the toes as far as comfortably possible.
- Extend the toes as far as comfortably possible.
- Each repetition of the sequence should take 1 to 3 seconds. Repeat as a continuous, controlled, fluid sequence 10 to 12 times.
- Repeat the sequence with the other foot.

breathe **Breathe evenly while performing the sequence.**

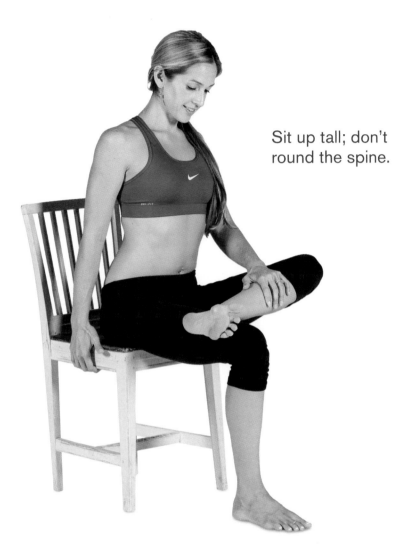

Sit up tall; don't round the spine.

▪ Sit in a chair, resting one ankle just above the opposite knee. Wiggle the toes as much as comfortably possible.

▪ Repeat as a continuous, controlled, fluid sequence 10 to 30 seconds.

▪ Repeat the sequence with the other foot.

breathe **Breathe evenly while performing the sequence.**

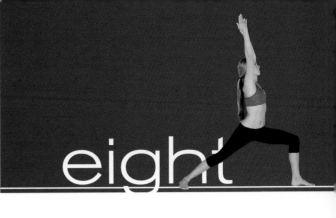

Multiregion Stretches

This chapter presents stretches that target multiple regions of the body at once. These stretches are more advanced than many of the other stretches in this book and are inspired by some of the world's most popular yoga poses. These stretches require both strength and flexibility and are designed to provide a multitude of energizing and functional benefits. Don't get discouraged if you can't do the stretches perfectly right away. Take your time; be patient with yourself. You'll find the stretches get easier each time you do them—and you might be surprised how much stronger you become.

Relax the neck and the shoulders.

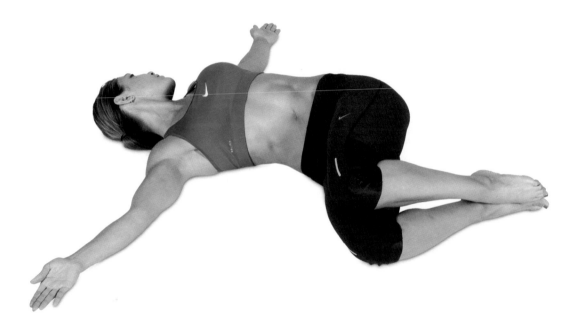

- Lie on the floor face up with the knees bent and the arms extended to the sides of the body at chest height. Rotate the hips and the knees to one side of the body as far as comfortably possible. Turn the head in the opposite direction of the hips and the knees.
- Hold the stretch for 10 to 30 seconds.
- Repeat the stretch on the other side.

 Exhale deeply while moving into the farthest point of the stretch; then breathe evenly while holding the stretch.

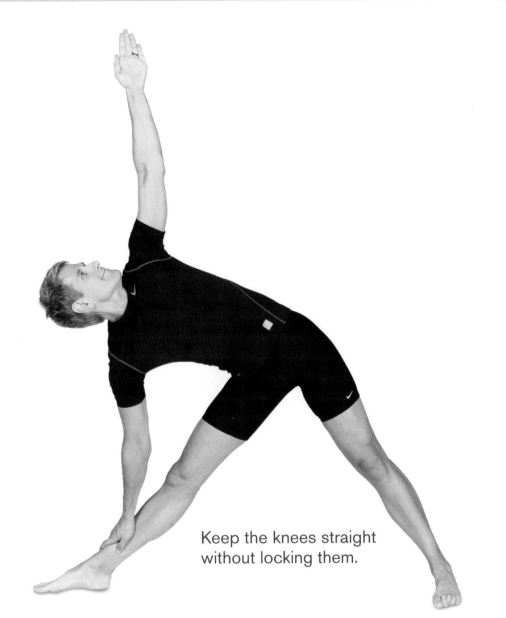

Keep the knees straight
without locking them.

- Stand with the feet about 3 feet (.9 m) apart with one foot and leg pointed forward and the other foot and leg turned out about 90 degrees. Bend toward the turned-out foot and leg and stretch the upper arm above the head. Rest the lower hand on the shin or the ankle. Turn the head to look toward the top hand.
- Hold the stretch for 10 to 30 seconds.
- Repeat the stretch on the other side.

Exhale deeply while moving into the farthest point of the stretch; then breathe evenly while holding the stretch.

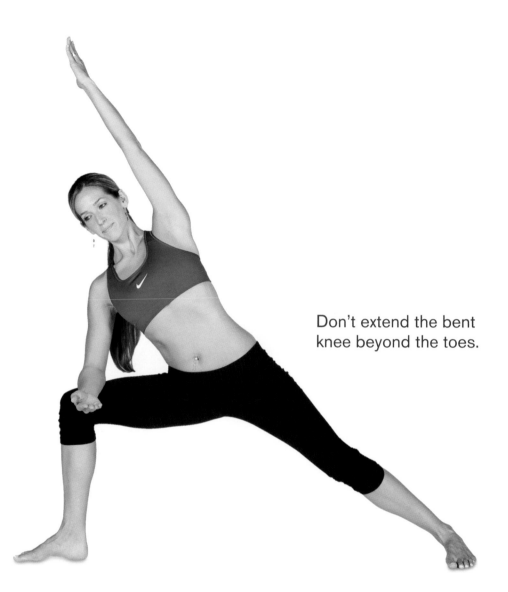

Don't extend the bent knee beyond the toes.

- Stand with the feet about 4 feet (1.2 m) apart with one foot pointed forward and the other foot and leg turned out about 90 degrees. Bend the knee of the turned-out leg and lean toward the same foot. Stretch the upper arm above the head so that it forms a straight line with the torso and the leg; rest the lower arm on the thigh.

- Hold the stretch for 10 to 30 seconds.

- Repeat the stretch on the other side.

 breathe **Exhale deeply while moving into the farthest point of the stretch; then breathe evenly while holding the stretch.**

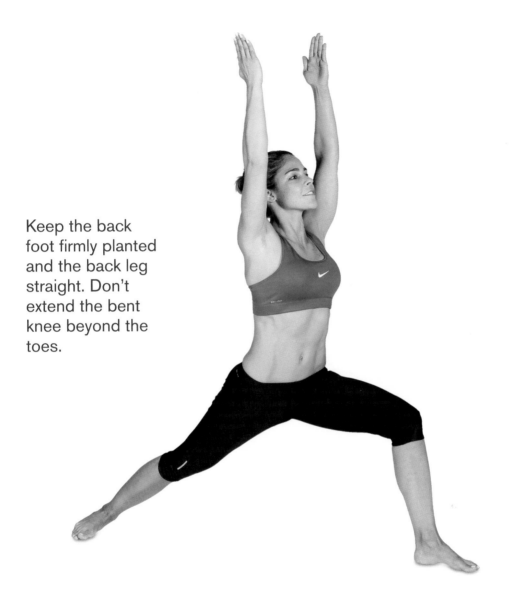

Keep the back foot firmly planted and the back leg straight. Don't extend the bent knee beyond the toes.

- Stand with the feet about 4 feet (1.2 m) apart with one foot pointed forward and the other foot and leg extended behind and turned out about 90 degrees. Bend the knee of the forward leg to 90 degrees. Raise both arms overhead with palms facing each other; rotate the upper body to face the direction of the bent knee.

- Hold the stretch for 10 to 30 seconds.

- Repeat the stretch on the other side.

breathe

Exhale deeply while moving into the farthest point of the stretch; then breathe evenly while holding the stretch.

Chair
Achilles tendon, soleus, gluteals, abdominals

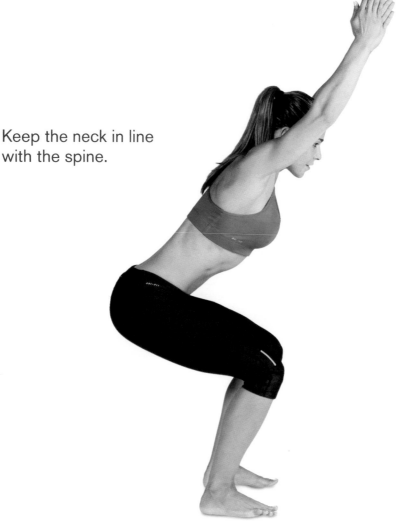

Keep the neck in line
with the spine.

■ Stand with the feet slightly apart. Bend the knees and lean the upper body
forward slightly. Drop the hips as if sitting in a chair.

■ Keep the palms slightly apart.

■ Hold the stretch for 10 to 30 seconds.

breathe

**Exhale deeply while moving into the farthest point of the
stretch; then breathe evenly while holding the stretch.**

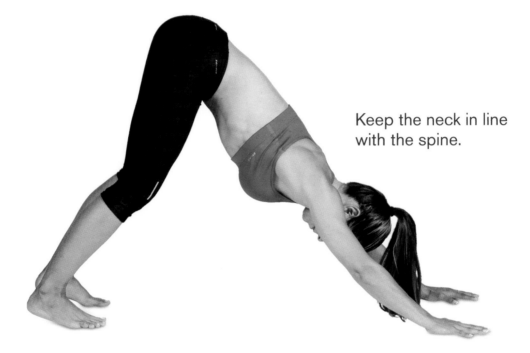

Keep the neck in line
with the spine.

▌ Kneel with the hands on the floor. Lift the tailbone and bring the knees off the
floor. Bring the shoulders and the head down. Keep the knees bent at first,
and then slowly bring the heels to the floor and straighten the knees. Lengthen
the spine as far as comfortably possible.

▌ Hold the stretch for 10 to 30 seconds.

breathe **Exhale deeply while moving into the farthest point of the
stretch; then breathe evenly while holding the stretch.**

Look straight ahead. Don't lift higher than is comfortable for the lower back.

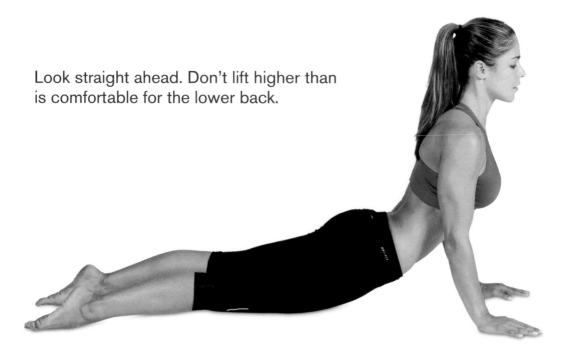

- Lie on the floor face down with the hands near the shoulders. Lift the body off the floor by pushing with the hands.
- Hold the stretch for 10 to 30 seconds.

 breathe **Exhale deeply while moving into the farthest point of the stretch; then breathe evenly while holding the stretch.**

Relax the neck and
the shoulders.

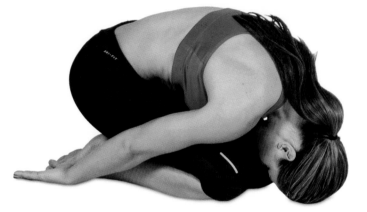

■ Kneel on the floor, sit back on the heels, and bring the forehead to the floor.
Rest the arms alongside the body with the palms facing up.

■ Hold the stretch for 10 to 30 seconds.

breathe **Exhale deeply while moving into the farthest point of the
stretch; then breathe evenly while holding the stretch.**

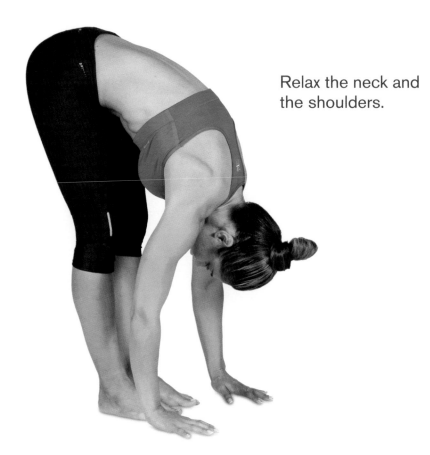

Relax the neck and
the shoulders.

- Standing with the feet together, raise the arms overhead. Bend forward at the hips and bring the nose toward the knees and the hands on (or toward) the floor.
- Hold the stretch for 10 to 30 seconds.

breathe **Exhale deeply while moving into the farthest point of the stretch; then breathe evenly while holding the stretch.**

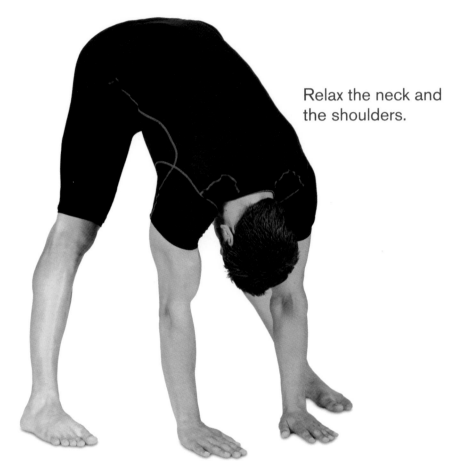

Relax the neck and the shoulders.

- ▮ Stand with the feet 3 to 4 feet (.9-1 m) apart with the feet facing forward. Bend forward at the hips and place the hands on (or toward) the floor in front of the feet.
- ▮ Hold the stretch for 10 to 30 seconds.

breathe **Exhale deeply while moving into the farthest point of the stretch; then breathe evenly while holding the stretch.**

Sitting Angular Leg Extension

Hamstrings, adductors, trunk extensors

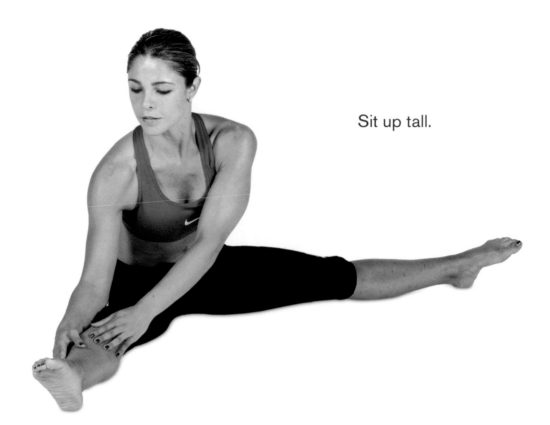

Sit up tall.

- Sit on the floor and spread the legs apart as far as comfortably possible. Bending forward at the hips, reach toward one ankle with both hands.
- Hold the stretch for 10 to 30 seconds.
- Repeat on the other side.

breathe   **Exhale deeply while moving into the farthest point of the stretch; then breathe evenly while holding the stretch.**

Dynamic Four-Legged Table

Biceps, hip flexors, deltoids, wrist flexors active

Keep the knees over the ankles and the shoulders over the hands.

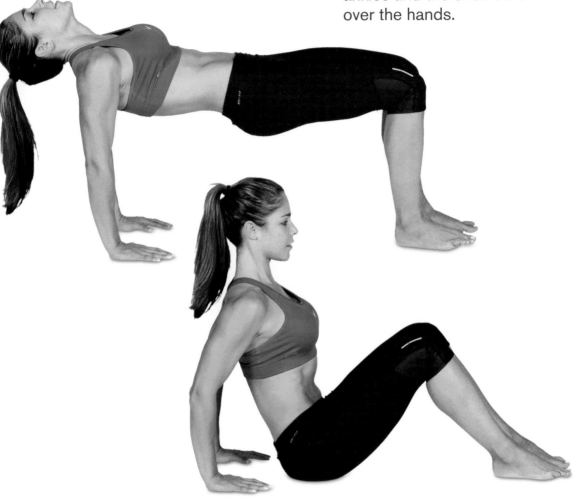

- Sit on the floor, extending the legs straight out in front with the knees bent. Keep the feet hip-width apart. Place the hands behind the body with the fingers facing forward.
- Lift the hips off the floor and try to place the knees, the hips, and the shoulders parallel to the floor. Keep the head in line with the spine, looking up.
- Release the stretch by returning to the start position.
- Each repetition of the sequence should take 1 to 3 seconds. Repeat as a continuous, controlled, fluid sequence 10 to 12 times.

 Exhale while lifting the hips off the floor; inhale each time the stretch is released.

163

Keep the shoulders over the
hands and the toes pointed.

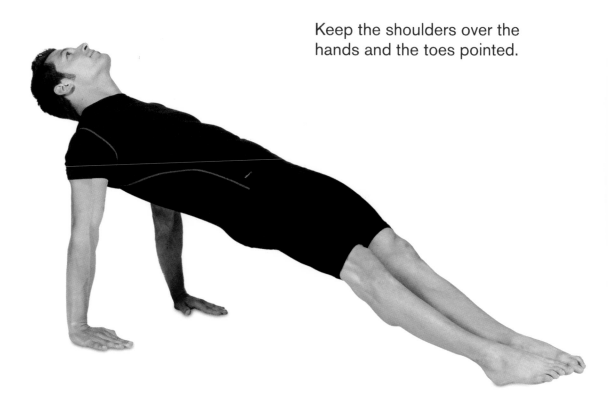

- Sit on the floor, extending the legs straight out in front. Place the hands behind the body with the fingers facing forward. Keeping the legs straight, lift the hips off the floor. The knees, the hips, and the shoulders should be in a straight line. Keep the head in line with the spine.

- Hold the stretch for 10 to 30 seconds.

breathe **Exhale deeply while moving into the farthest point of the stretch; then breathe evenly while holding the stretch.**

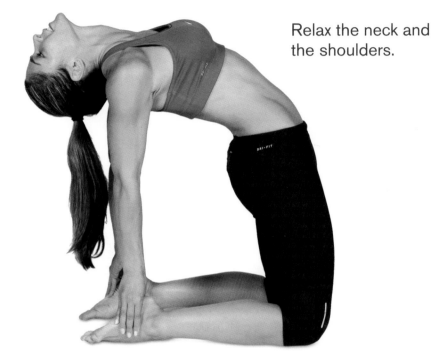

Relax the neck and
the shoulders.

- Begin in an upright kneeling position on the floor. Reach back and grasp the ankles with the same-side hands. Allowing the head to slowly lower, arch and lean back as far as comfortably possible.
- Hold the stretch for 10 to 30 seconds.

breathe

Exhale deeply while moving into the farthest point of the stretch; then breathe evenly while holding the stretch.

Dynamic Bow

Abdominals, deltoids, hip flexors

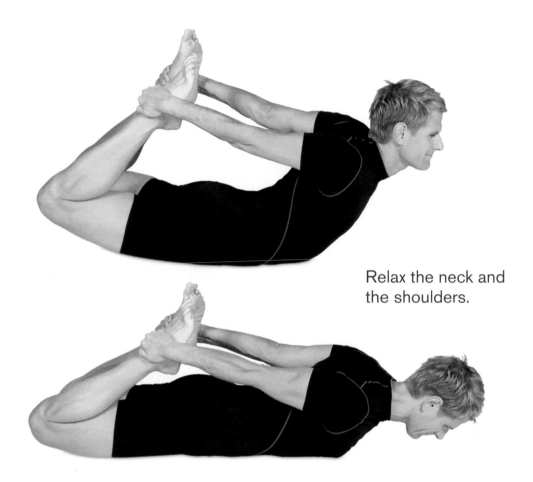

Relax the neck and the shoulders.

- Lie on the floor face down. Bend the knees and reach behind and grasp both ankles with the same-side hands.
- Slowly raise the legs by pulling the ankles up and raising the knees off the floor while simultaneously raising the chest off the floor. Tilt the head back slightly.
- Release the stretch by returning to the start position.
- Each repetition of the sequence should take 1 to 3 seconds. Repeat as a continuous, controlled, fluid sequence 10 to 12 times.

 Exhale while raising the ankles, the knees, and the chest off the floor; inhale each time the stretch is released.

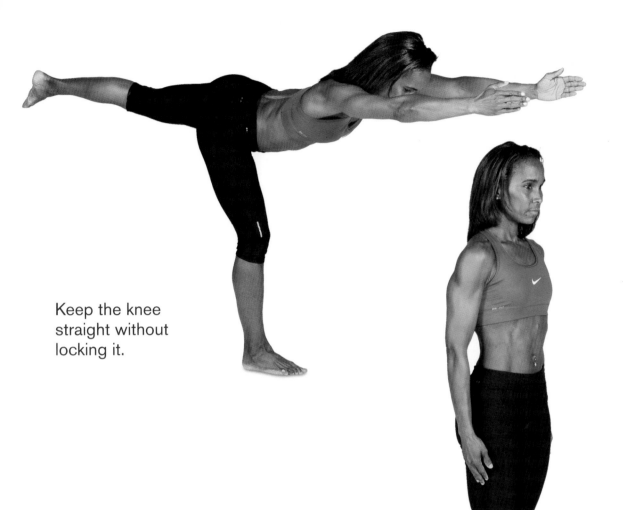

Keep the knee
straight without
locking it.

- Stand with the feet together.
- Pivot forward at the hips, extending the arms straight alongside the head and lifting one leg behind the body parallel to the floor.
- Release the stretch by returning to the start position.
- Each repetition of the sequence should take 1 to 3 seconds. Repeat as a continuous, controlled, fluid sequence 10 to 12 times.
- Repeat the stretch with the other leg.

breathe

Exhale while pivoting forward at the hips; inhale each time the stretch is released.

Eagle

Rhomboids (middle back), gluteals

Relax the neck and
the shoulders.

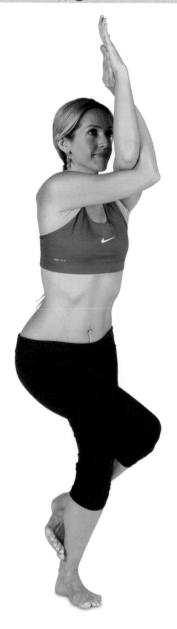

- Stand with the feet together. Bend one knee, raise the knee across the other thigh, and wrap the foot around the supporting leg. Cross the same-side arm as the lifted leg in front of the other arm and place the palms together, the fingers pointing up.
- Hold the stretch for 10 to 30 seconds.
- Repeat the stretch with the other leg and arm.

 Exhale deeply while moving into the farthest point of the stretch; then breathe evenly while holding the stretch.

Relax the neck and the shoulders.

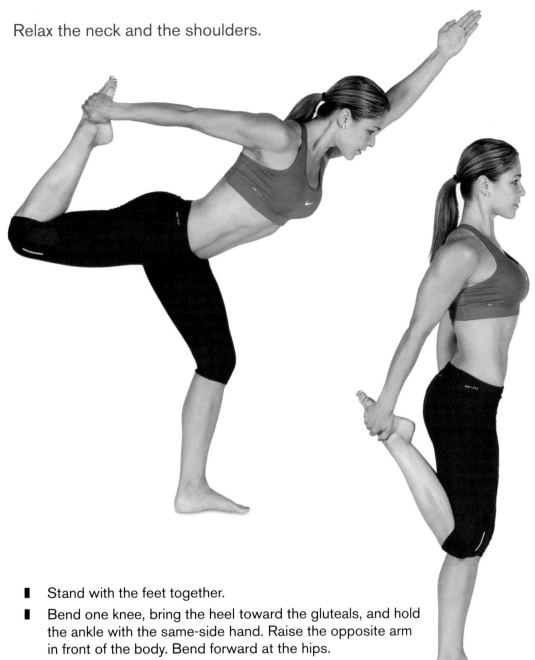

- Stand with the feet together.
- Bend one knee, bring the heel toward the gluteals, and hold the ankle with the same-side hand. Raise the opposite arm in front of the body. Bend forward at the hips.
- Release the stretch by returning to the start position.
- Each repetition of the sequence should take 1 to 3 seconds. Repeat as a continuous, controlled, fluid sequence 10 to 12 times.
- Repeat the stretch with the other leg.

breathe **Exhale while bending forward at the hips; inhale each time the stretch is released.**

Dynamic Grasshopper
Abdominals, hip flexors

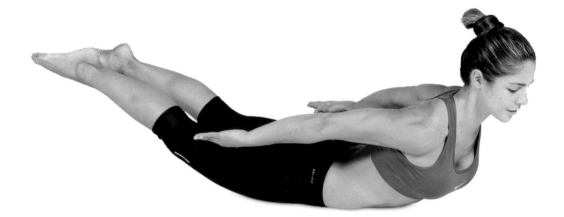

Don't lift higher than comfortably possible.

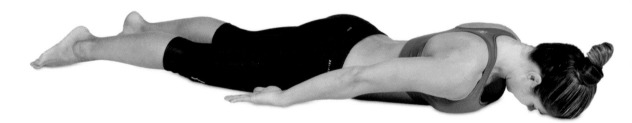

- Lie on the floor face down. Rest the arms alongside the body with the palms facing up.
- Raise the head, the chest, and the legs off the floor as high as comfortably possible. Tilt the head back.
- Release the stretch by returning to the start position.
- Each repetition of the sequence should take 1 to 3 seconds. Repeat as a continuous, controlled, fluid sequence 10 to 12 times.

breathe

Exhale while raising the head, the chest, and the legs off the floor; inhale each time the stretch is released.

Keep the knees straight
without locking them.

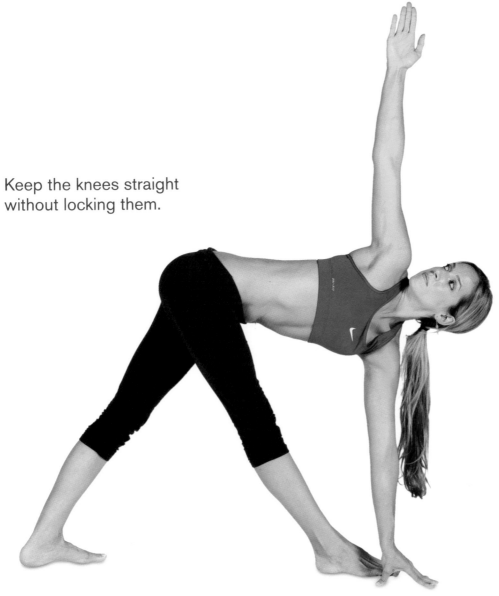

- Stand with the feet about 3-4 feet (.9-1 m) apart with one foot pointed forward and the other foot and the leg turned out about 90 degrees. Raise both arms to the sides at chest height, rotate the upper body, and face the forward-pointing foot. Bend forward from the hips and rotate the torso to the outside of the thigh of the forward-facing foot. Reach the lower hand toward the floor or the shin of the forward-facing foot. Turn the head and look up toward the top hand.
- Hold the stretch for 10 to 30 seconds.
- Repeat the stretch on the other side.

breathe
Exhale deeply while moving into the farthest point of the stretch; then breathe evenly while holding the stretch.

Cow Face

Triceps, deltoid (front shoulder), quadriceps

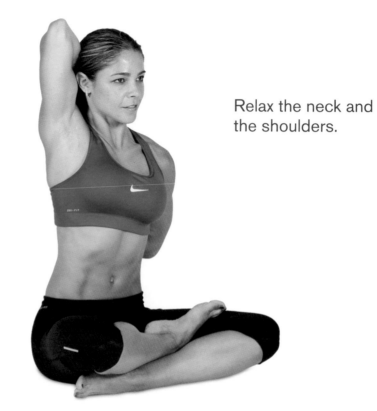

Relax the neck and the shoulders.

- Sit in a crossed-leg position, one leg over the other leg, with the feet as close to the body as comfortably possible. Raise one hand over the head and bend the elbow. Reach behind the back with the other hand; clasp fingers of the two hands together.
- Hold the stretch for 10 to 30 seconds.
- Repeat on the other side.

 Exhale deeply while moving into the farthest point of the stretch; then breathe evenly while holding the stretch.

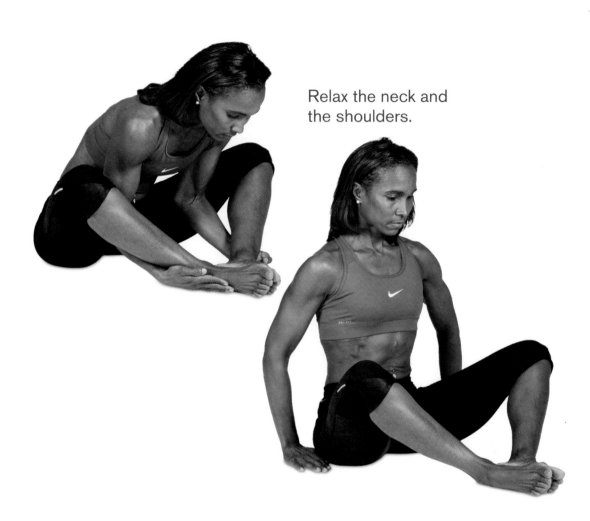

Relax the neck and
the shoulders.

- Sit on the floor; bend the knees and bring the soles of the feet together.
- Drop the chest between the legs toward the floor. Place the hands under the ankles and hold the feet.
- Release the stretch by returning to the start position.
- Each repetition of the sequence should take 1 to 3 seconds. Repeat as a continuous, controlled, fluid sequence 10 to 12 times.

breathe **Exhale while dropping the chest toward the floor; inhale each
time the stretch is released.**

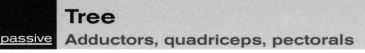

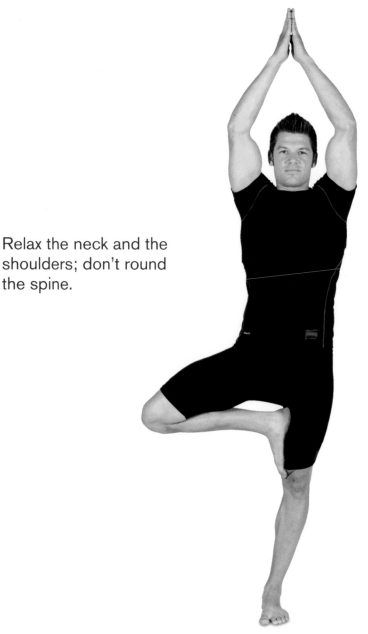

Relax the neck and the shoulders; don't round the spine.

- Stand with the feet together. Bend one knee, open the hip to the side, and place the sole of the foot on the inside of the opposite thigh as high up as comfortably possible. Extend the arms overhead; bring the palms of the hands together above the body.

- Hold the stretch for 10 to 30 seconds.

- Repeat the stretch with the other leg.

 Exhale deeply while moving into the farthest point of the stretch; then breathe evenly while holding the stretch.

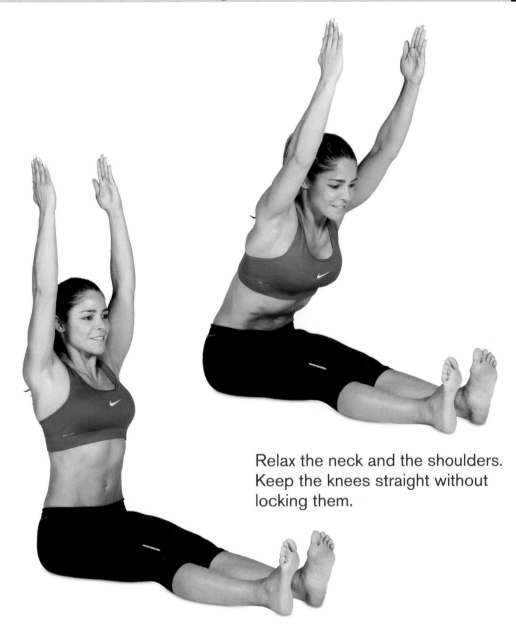

Relax the neck and the shoulders.
Keep the knees straight without
locking them.

- Sit on the floor, extending the legs in front of the body; extend the arms above the head.
- Slowly move the upper body toward the legs, pivoting at the hips. Bring the head as close to the knees as comfortably possible.
- Release the stretch by returning to the start position.
- Each repetition of the sequence should take 1 to 3 seconds. Repeat as a continuous, controlled, fluid sequence 10 to 12 times.

 Exhale while moving the upper body toward the legs; inhale each time the stretch is released.

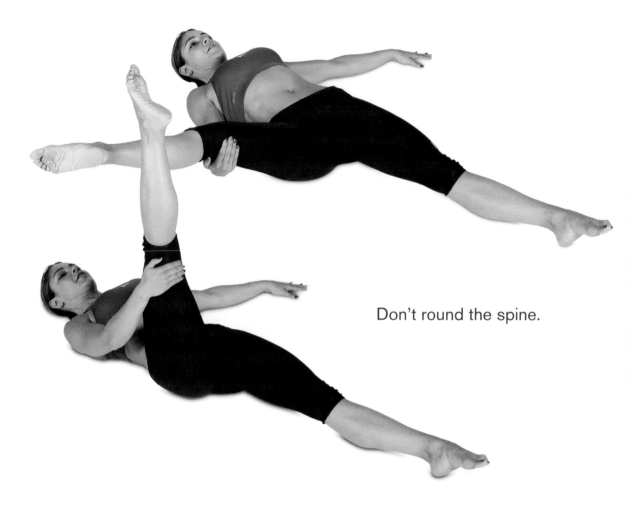

Don't round the spine.

- ▌ Lie on the floor face up.
- ▌ Lift one leg up and bring it toward the body, keeping the leg straight. Hold the foot, or outside of the lower leg, with the same-side hand. Bring the leg out to the side as far as comfortably possible.
- ▌ Release the stretch by returning to the start position.
- ▌ Each repetition of the sequence should take 1 to 3 seconds. Repeat as a continuous, controlled, fluid sequence 10 to 12 times.
- ▌ Repeat the stretch with the other leg.

breathe **Exhale while moving the leg out to the side; inhale each time the stretch is released.**

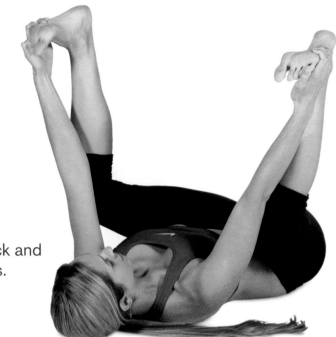

Relax the neck and the shoulders.

■ Lie on the floor face up. Bend the knees toward the chest and hold the toes or outside of the feet with the hands. Open the legs and bring the knees toward the floor.

■ Hold the stretch for 10 to 30 seconds.

breathe **Exhale deeply while moving into the farthest point of the stretch; then breathe evenly while holding the stretch.**

177

Half Moon

Adductors, pectorals

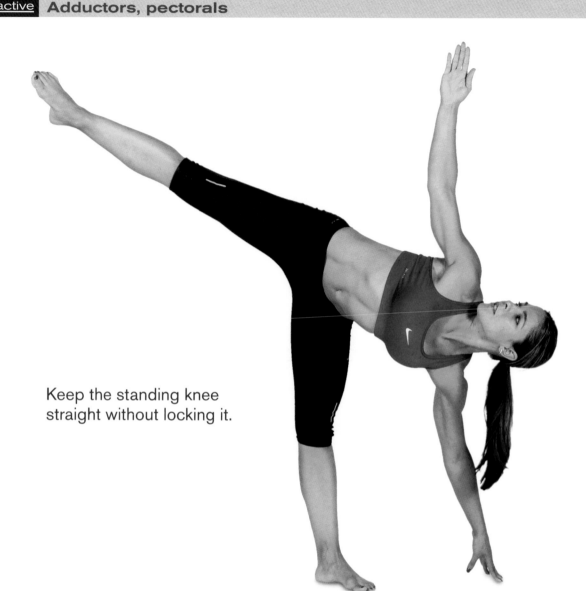

Keep the standing knee
straight without locking it.

■ Stand with the feet together. Extend the arms out to the sides of the body at
chest height. Turn one foot perpendicular to the body and lean to the same
side while simultaneously raising the other leg off the floor. Place the same-
side hand of the standing foot on the floor, keep the top shoulder, the hip, the
knee, and the ankle in line, and point the raised foot forward. Turn the head
and look up at the top hand.

■ Hold the stretch for 10 to 30 seconds.

■ Repeat on the other side.

 **Exhale deeply while moving into the farthest point of the
stretch; then breathe evenly while holding the stretch.**

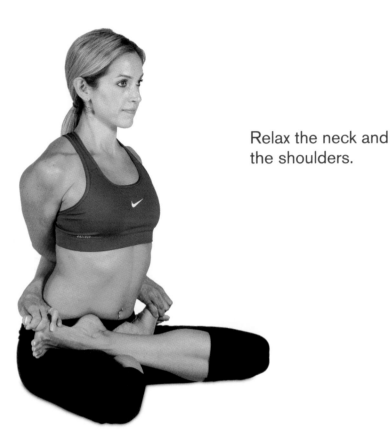

Relax the neck and the shoulders.

■ Sit in a crossed-leg position with each foot resting on top of the opposite thigh as close to the body as comfortably possible. Sitting up tall, reach around and behind the back with both hands to grasp the toes of the same-side foot.

■ Hold the stretch for 10 to 30 seconds.

breathe **Exhale deeply while moving into the farthest point of the stretch; then breathe evenly while holding the stretch.**

Frog

Adductors, tibialis anterior

Sit lightly
on the feet.

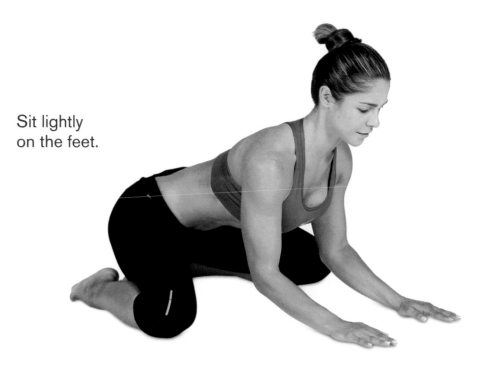

- Kneel on the floor and sit back on the heels. Place the palms of the hands on the floor in front of the knees. Open the legs as far as comfortably possible.
- Hold the stretch for 10 to 30 seconds.

 Exhale deeply while moving into the farthest point of the stretch; then breathe evenly while holding the stretch.

Dynamic Leg Cradle
Gluteals, piriformis

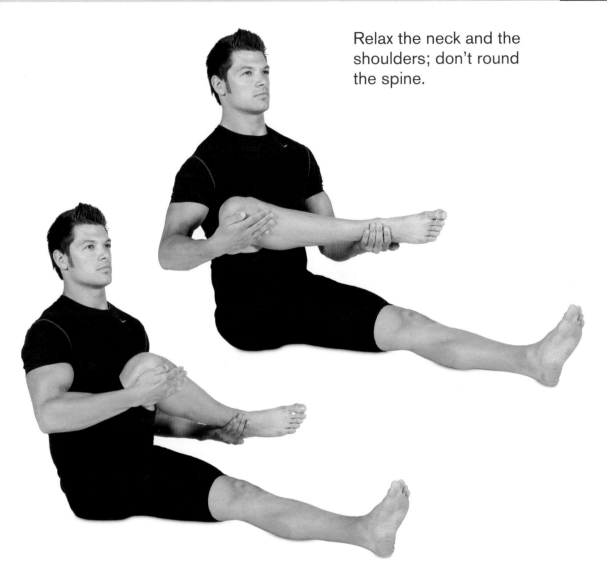

Relax the neck and the shoulders; don't round the spine.

- Sit on the floor, extending the legs out in front of the body; bend one knee and place the foot on the floor.
- Hold the outside of the bent knee with the same-side arm; hold the outside of the ankle with the opposite arm. Move the leg in a clockwise (or counterclockwise) circular motion toward the opposite shoulder.
- Release the stretch by returning to the start position.
- Each repetition of the sequence should take 1 to 3 seconds. Repeat as a continuous, controlled, fluid sequence 10 to 12 times.
- Repeat the sequence with the other leg.

 Exhale while moving the leg in a circular motion; inhale each time the stretch is released.

Dynamic Half-Circle

Adductors, latissimus dorsi, lateral trunk flexors

Don't lean forward or back.

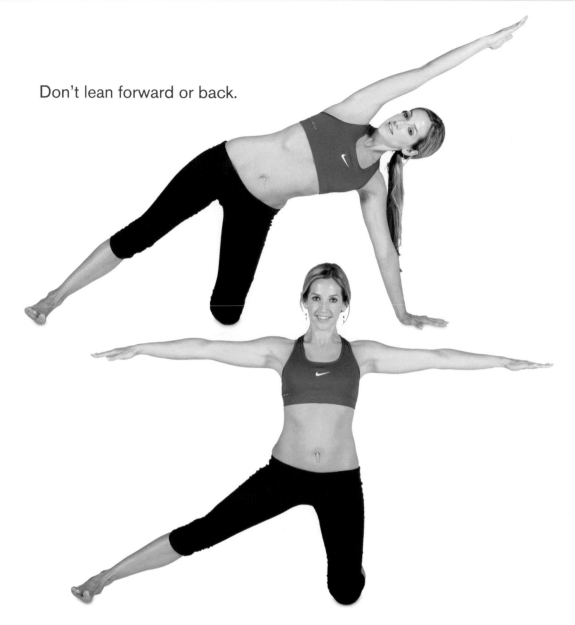

- Kneel on the floor, extending one leg straight out to the side of the body.
- Lean to the side of the kneeling leg; place the same-side hand on the floor. Reach overhead and across the body with the opposite arm while bending the torso toward the lower arm.
- Release the stretch by returning to the start position.
- Each repetition of the sequence should take 1 to 3 seconds. Repeat as a continuous, controlled, fluid sequence 10 to 12 times.
- Repeat on the other side.

breathe **Exhale while leaning to one side; inhale each time the stretch is released.**

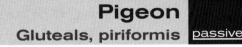

Relax the neck and the shoulders;
don't round the spine.

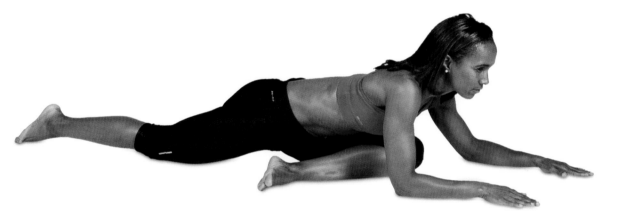

- Sit on the floor with the legs extended in front of the body as wide as comfortably possible. Rotate the torso toward one leg; bend the knee of the same leg to 90 degrees. Place both hands on the floor in front of the bent knee. Lower the chest toward the inner thigh of the bent knee and bring the straight leg behind the body, resting the outside of the leg on the floor.
- Hold the stretch for 10 to 30 seconds.
- Repeat the sequence with the other leg.

 Exhale deeply while moving into the farthest point of the stretch; then breathe evenly while holding the stretch.

One-Legged King Pigeon

Gluteals, piriformis, abdominals, hip flexors, quadriceps

Point the elbows toward the ceiling. Don't extend beyond the point that is comfortable for the lower back.

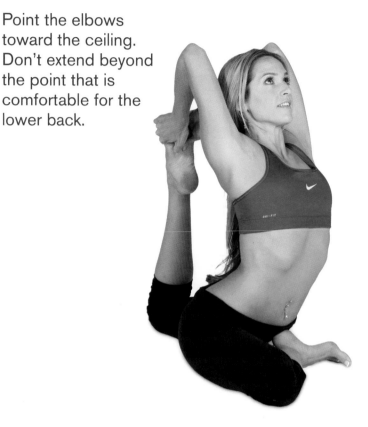

- Sit on the floor with the legs extended in front of the body as wide as comfortably possible. Rotate the torso toward one leg, bend the knee of the same leg to 90 degrees. Bring the straight leg behind the body, resting the front of the thigh on the floor, and sit up tall. Bend the knee of the straight leg, arch and lean back as far as comfortably possible, and reach behind and grasp the foot with both hands.

- Hold the stretch for 10 to 30 seconds.

- Repeat on the other leg.

Exhale deeply while moving into the farthest point of the stretch, then continue to breathe evenly while holding the stretch.

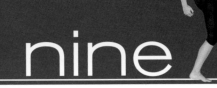

Sport Mobility Stretches

This chapter features stretches designed to improve athletic range of motion and mobility. All of these dynamic stretches can be used to warm up or to prepare for performance-oriented, multidirectional activities, such as soccer, tennis, basketball, and volleyball. The stretches emphasize bending, reaching, and rotating using sport-inspired movement patterns. Many of the stretches also improve agility, coordination, and balance.

Dynamic Straight-Leg Pendulum
Hamstrings, hip flexors

Relax the neck and
the shoulders. Let the
arms swing naturally.

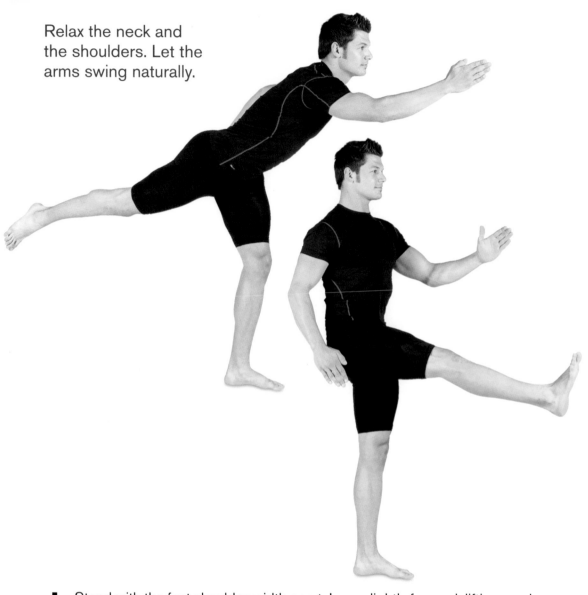

- Stand with the feet shoulder-width apart. Lean slightly forward, lifting one leg up behind the body as high as comfortably possible, keeping the leg straight.
- Bring the upper body to an upright position. Raise the lifted leg forward as high as comfortably possible, keeping the leg straight.
- Each repetition of the sequence should take 1 to 2 seconds and should be performed with controlled momentum. Pause 1 second between repetitions. Repeat the sequence 10 to 12 times.
- Repeat the sequence on the other leg.

breathe   **Breathe evenly while performing the sequence.**

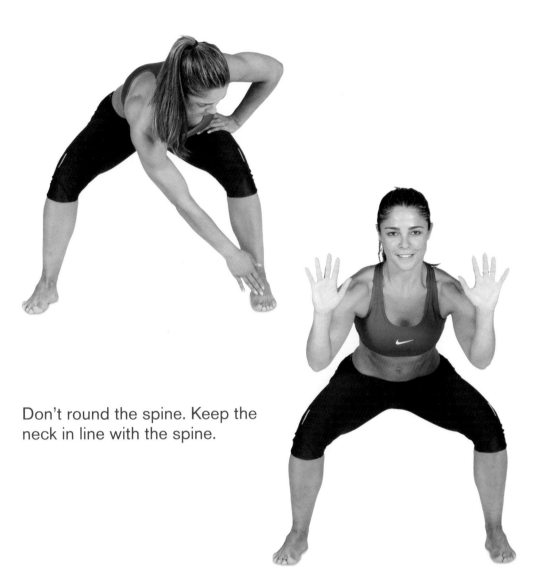

Don't round the spine. Keep the neck in line with the spine.

▌ Stand with the feet and the legs in a wide squat position. Reach down and touch the inside of one foot with the opposite hand; then immediately touch the inside of the other foot with the other hand. Rotate the upper body slightly with each foot-touch. Then quickly bring the feet together and slide laterally to one side into another squat.

▌ Repeat the sequence leading with the opposite hand.

▌ Slide laterally back to the start position.

▌ Each repetition of the sequence should take 1 to 3 seconds and should be performed with controlled momentum. Repeat the sequence 10 to 12 times.

breathe   **Breathe evenly while performing the sequence.**

Dynamic Leg Kick

Hamstrings, trunk extensors (lower back), gluteals

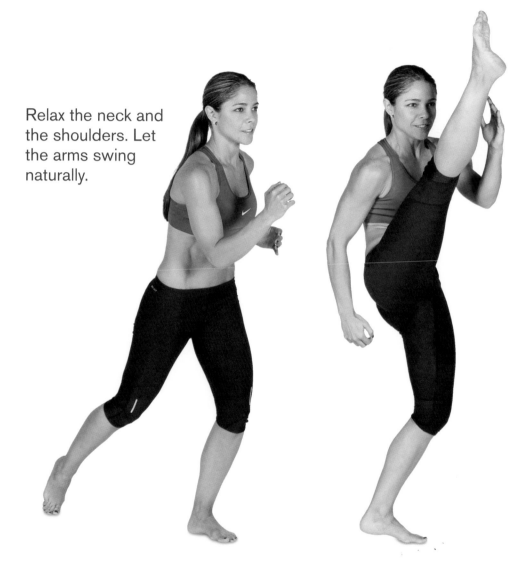

Relax the neck and the shoulders. Let the arms swing naturally.

- Stand with the feet shoulder-width apart. Leap forward with one leg to perform a straight-leg kick with the other leg as high as comfortably possible.
- Return to the start position.
- Each repetition of the sequence should take 1 to 2 seconds and should be performed with controlled momentum. Pause 1 second between repetitions. Repeat the sequence 10 to 12 times.
- Repeat the sequence on the other leg.

breathe **Breathe evenly while performing the sequence.**

Dynamic Cross-Knee Squat

Abductors, gluteals, hamstrings, trunk extensors (lower back) active

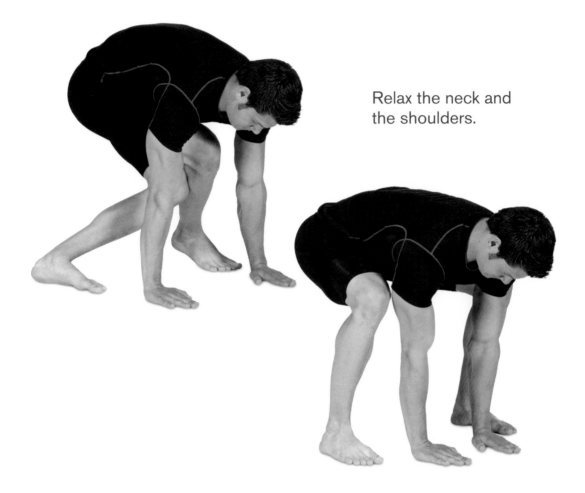

Relax the neck and the shoulders.

▮ Stand with the feet in a wide squat position. Lift one leg, bend the knee, and move the knee across the body as far as comfortably possible, rotating the hips and torso while keeping the chest and the shoulders facing forward.

▮ Repeat the sequence with the other leg.

▮ Leaning forward, bend the knees and reach down to place the palms of the hands on (or toward) the floor.

▮ Return to the start position.

▮ Each repetition of the sequence should take 1 to 3 seconds and should be performed with controlled momentum. Pause 1 second between repetitions. Repeat the sequence 10 to 12 times.

breathe **Breathe evenly while performing the sequence.**

Dynamic Squat Twist Reach

Hamstrings, gluteals, abdominals, pectorals, deltoids

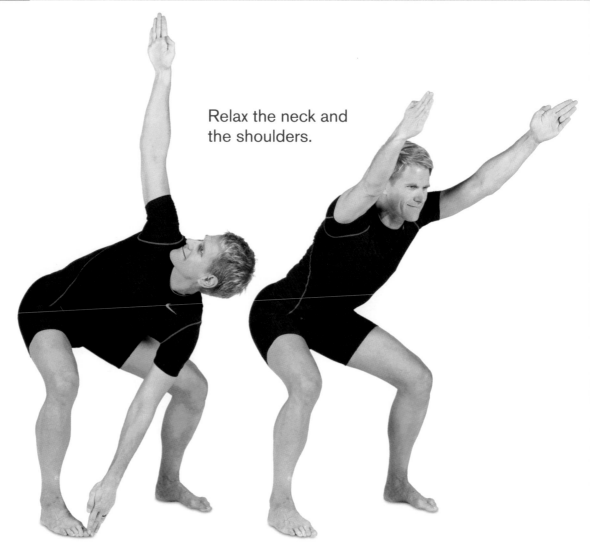

Relax the neck and
the shoulders.

- Stand with the feet shoulder-width apart. Squat down as far as comfortably possible.
- Rotate the upper body and touch the outside of one ankle with the opposite hand while reaching behind and above the body with the other hand. Turn the head to look up at the hand above the body.
- Return to the start position.
- Extend both hands over the head while slightly arching the back.
- Repeat the sequence on the other side.
- Each repetition of the sequence should take 1 to 3 seconds and should be performed with controlled momentum. Pause 1 second between repetitions. Repeat the sequence 10 to 12 times.

breathe **Breathe evenly while performing the sequence.**

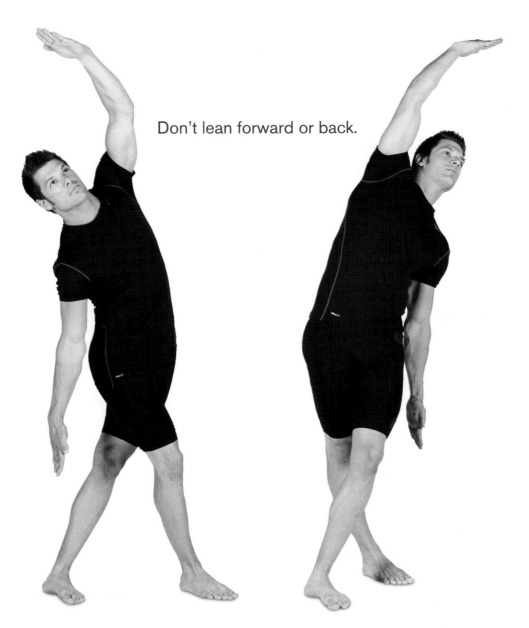

Don't lean forward or back.

■ Stand with the feet shoulder-width apart. Cross one leg in front of the other leg; reach over the head and across the body with the opposite arm while reaching toward the foot with the lower arm.

■ Return to the start position and repeat the sequence on the other side.

■ Each repetition of the sequence should take 1 to 2 seconds and should be performed with controlled momentum. Pause 1 second between repetitions. Repeat the sequence 10 to 12 times.

breathe **Breathe evenly while performing the sequence.**

Dynamic Lunge and Push Back

Hip flexors, gluteals

Don't extend the front knee
beyond the toes.

▮ Stand with the feet shoulder-width apart. Take a giant
step forward into a deep lunge position with the front
knee bent and the back leg straight. Lean forward and
place the hands on the floor on either side of the front
leg. Then push back to the start position using the front
leg and both arms.

▮ Each repetition of the sequence should take 1 to 3 seconds and should be
performed with controlled momentum. Pause 1 second between repetitions.
Repeat the sequence 10 to 12 times.

▮ Repeat the sequence with the other leg.

breathe   **Breathe evenly while performing the sequence.**

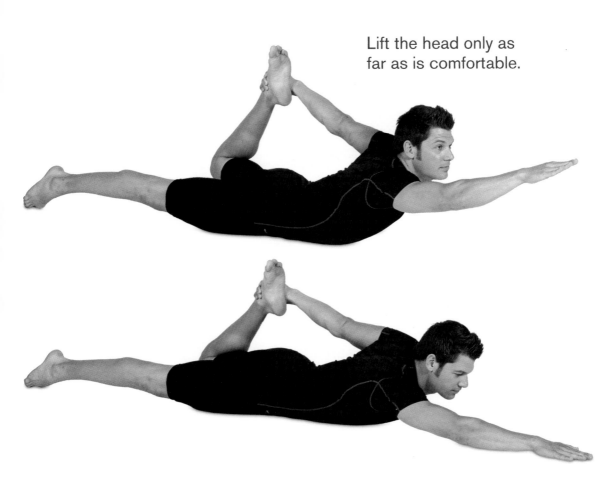

Lift the head only as
far as is comfortable.

- Lie on the floor face down. Bend one knee and bring the heel of the foot toward the gluteals while lifting the shoulders off the ground. Reach back toward the foot with the same-side hand and extend the opposite arm straight out in front of the body.

- Return to the start position and repeat on the other side.

- Each repetition of the sequence should take 1 to 3 seconds and should be performed with controlled momentum. Pause 1 second between repetitions. Repeat the sequence 10 to 12 times.

breathe **Breathe evenly while performing the sequence.**

Dynamic Lunge and Twist

Adductors, abdominals, trunk extensors

Relax the neck and the shoulders.
Don't extend the knee beyond
the toes.

■ Stand with the feet about 4 feet (1 m) apart. Bend one knee while reaching toward the same-side foot with the opposite hand.

■ Repeat on the other side; then return to the start position.

■ Raise arms out in front of the body at chest height with the elbows bent; twist the arms and torso to one side, then to the other side, and then back to center.

■ Each repetition of the sequence should take 2 to 4 seconds and should be performed with controlled momentum. Pause 1 second between repetitions. Repeat the sequence 10 to 12 times.

breathe **Breathe evenly while performing the sequence.**

Relax the neck and the shoulders.

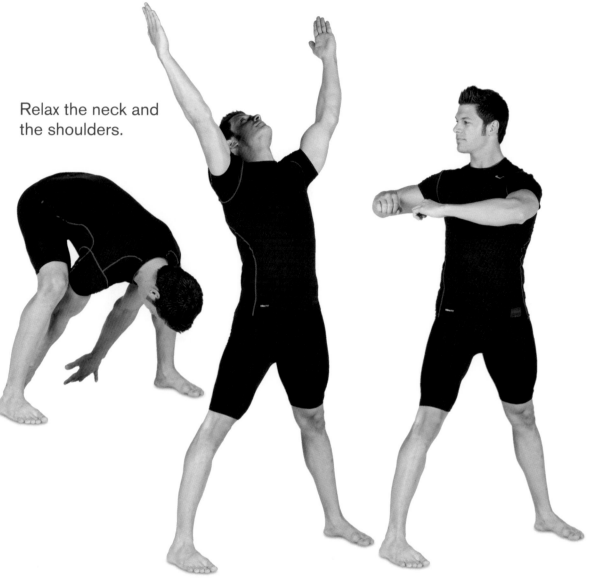

- Stand with the feet in a wide squat position. Reach between the feet with both hands and touch the floor as far back as comfortably possible. Reach up over the head with both arms and arch the back slightly.

- Return to the start position.

- Raise the arms out in front of the body at chest height with the elbows bent; twist the arms and the torso to one side, then to the other side, and then back to center.

- Each repetition of the sequence should take 2 to 4 seconds and should be performed with controlled momentum. Pause 1 second between repetitions. Repeat the sequence 10 to 12 times.

breathe **Breathe evenly while performing the sequence.**

Dynamic Knee Circle Twist

Gluteals, adductors, abductors, trunk extensors, abdominals

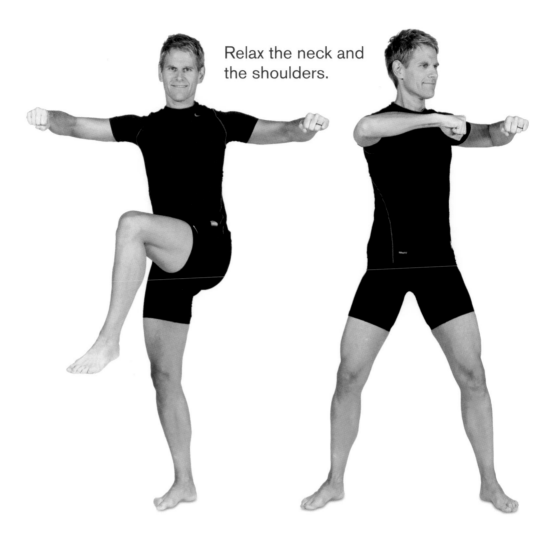

Relax the neck and the shoulders.

- Stand with the feet slightly more than shoulder-width apart. Lift one leg, bend the knee, and move the leg across the body in a large circular pattern.

- Return to the start position and repeat the sequence on the other side.

- Raise arms out in front of the body at chest height with the elbows bent; twist the arms and the torso to one side, then to the other side, and then back to center.

- Each repetition of the sequence should take 2 to 4 seconds and should be performed with controlled momentum. Pause 1 second between repetitions. Repeat the sequence 10 to 12 times.

breathe **Breathe evenly while performing the sequence.**

Dynamic Child's Pose and Camel

Quadriceps, hip flexors, abdominals, deltoids, pectorals

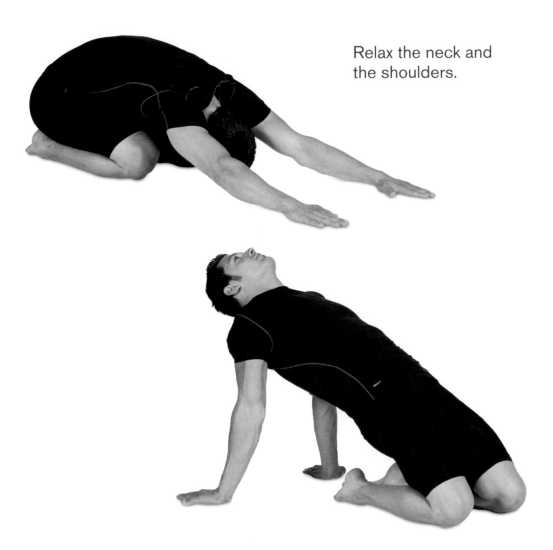

Relax the neck and the shoulders.

- Kneel on the floor. Place the hands in front of the body on the floor and sit back on the heels. Drop the chest toward the thighs as far as comfortably possible.
- Lift the upper body off the chest into an upright position. Lean back and reach behind the body to (or toward) the feet with both hands while pushing the hips forward.
- Return to the start position.
- Each repetition of the sequence should take 2 to 4 seconds and should be performed with controlled momentum. Pause 1 second between repetitions. Repeat the sequence 10 to 12 times.

breathe **Breathe evenly while performing the sequence.**

Dynamic Hip Swivel and Chest Lift

Abductors, abdominals, hip flexors

Lift the head only as
far as is comfortable.

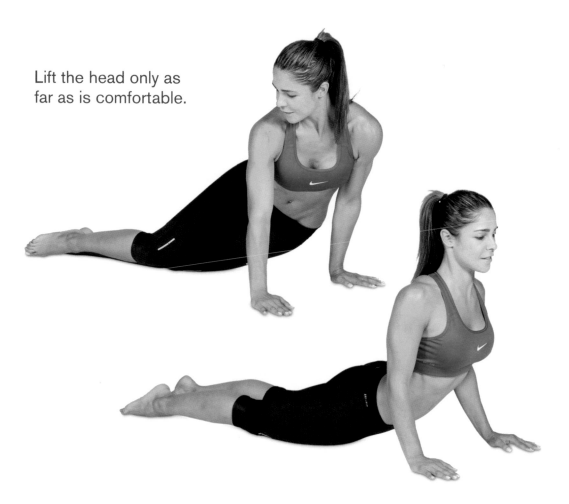

- Position on the floor on the hands and the knees. Shift the body to one side; lower the same-side hip to (or toward) the floor, pivoting on the knees.
- Return to the center. Repeat on the other side.
- Move the hands slightly forward and lower both hips to the floor while lifting the chest up and arching the back.
- Each repetition of the sequence should take 5 to 7 seconds and should be performed with controlled momentum. Pause 1 second between repetitions. Repeat the sequence 10 to 12 times.

breathe **Breathe evenly while performing the sequence.**

Dynamic Roll and Reach

Hamstrings, trunk extensors (lower back), gluteals

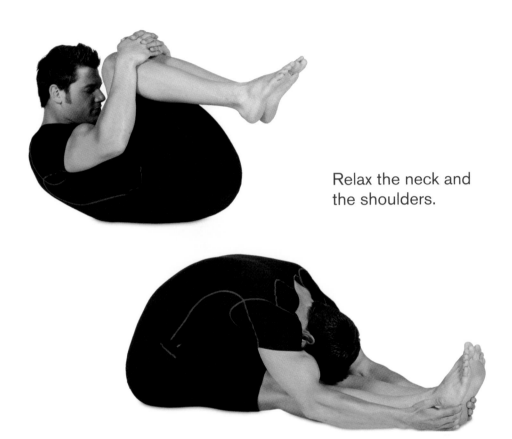

Relax the neck and the shoulders.

∎ Sit on the floor with the knees bent and the thighs close to the chest. Hold the shins with the hands. Keeping the chin tucked, push off with the toes and roll back gently until the shoulder blades touch the floor. Immediately roll back up into a seated position with the legs extended straight in front of the body and the arms reaching forward. Move the chest as close to the thighs as comfortably possible.

∎ Return to the start position.

∎ Each repetition of the sequence should take 2 to 4 seconds and should be performed with controlled momentum. Pause 1 second between repetitions. Repeat the sequence 10 to 12 times.

breathe **Breathe evenly while performing the sequence.**

Dynamic Squat Twist and Hinge

Hamstrings, gluteals, trunk extensors, abdominals

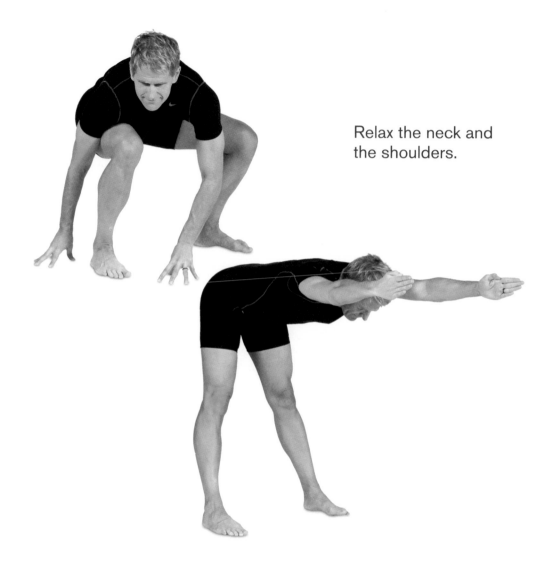

Relax the neck and the shoulders.

- Stand with the feet in a wide squat position. Bend the knees, rotate the upper body slightly, and place one hand on the floor in front of the body and one hand on the floor behind the body.

- Return to the start position and repeat on the other side.

- Extend the arms directly overhead and lean forward, hinging from the hips until the upper body is parallel to the floor.

- Return to the start position.

- Each repetition of the sequence should take 2 to 4 seconds and should be performed with controlled momentum. Pause 1 second between repetitions. Repeat the sequence 10 to 12 times.

breathe **Breathe evenly while performing the sequence.**

Dynamic Knee Lift and Leg Back

Hip flexors, gluteals, hamstrings <u>active</u>

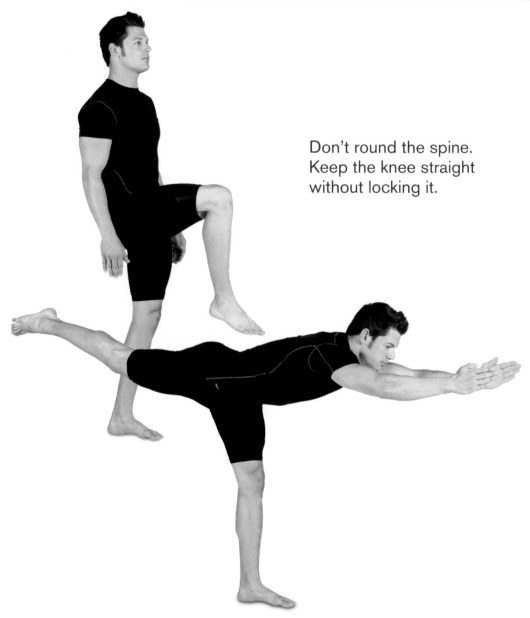

Don't round the spine. Keep the knee straight without locking it.

- Stand with the feet shoulder-width apart. Bend one knee and lift it in front of the body as high as comfortably possible. Lower the knee and lift the same leg behind the body (keeping the leg straight) while leaning forward and extending the arms alongside the ears.

- Return to the start position.

- Repeat the sequence with the other leg.

- Each repetition of the sequence should take 2 to 4 seconds and should be performed with controlled momentum. Pause 1 second between repetitions. Repeat the sequence 10 to 12 times.

breathe **Breathe evenly while performing the sequence.**

Dynamic Lateral Reach Slide

Adductors, abdominals, trunk extensors

Don't lean forward
or back.

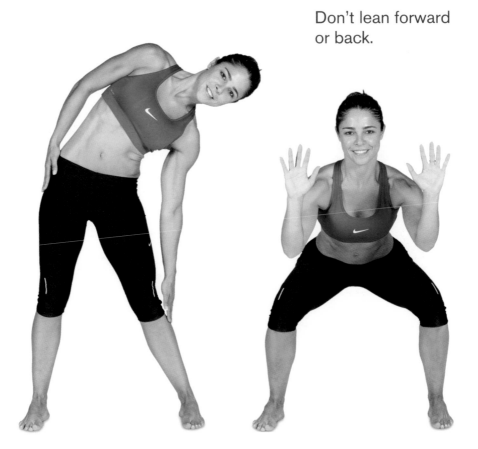

- Stand with the feet in a wide squat position. Reach down the side of one leg toward the outside of the same-leg foot while bending the torso to the same side.
- Return to the start position and repeat on the other side.
- Quickly bring the feet together and slide laterally to one side into another squat.
- Repeat the sequence leading with the opposite hand, and then slide laterally back to the start position.
- Each repetition of the sequence should take 2 to 4 seconds and should be performed with controlled momentum. Pause 1 second between repetitions. Repeat the sequence 10 to 12 times.

 Breathe evenly while performing the sequence.

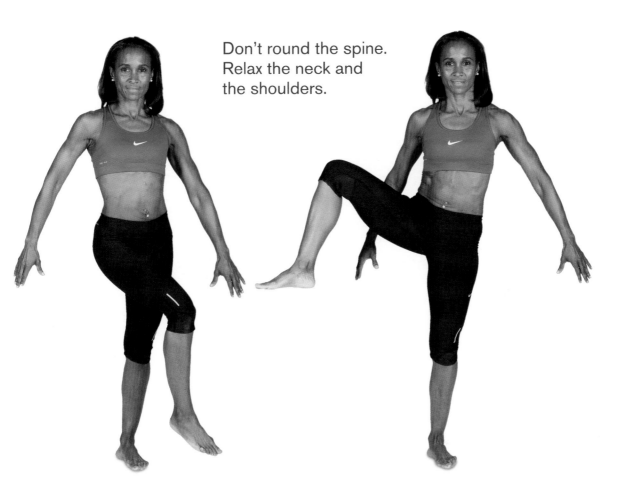

Don't round the spine. Relax the neck and the shoulders.

- Stand with the feet together. Bend one knee and lift it in front of the body. Move the knee in a figure-8 pattern, rotating through the hip.
- Return to the start position and repeat with the other leg.
- Each repetition of the sequence should take 2 to 3 seconds and should be performed with controlled momentum. Pause 1 second between repetitions. Repeat the sequence 10 to 12 times.

breathe **Breathe evenly while performing the sequence.**

Dynamic Knee Bend and Hug
Quadriceps, hamstrings, hip flexors, gluteals

Don't arch the back. Don't round the spine.

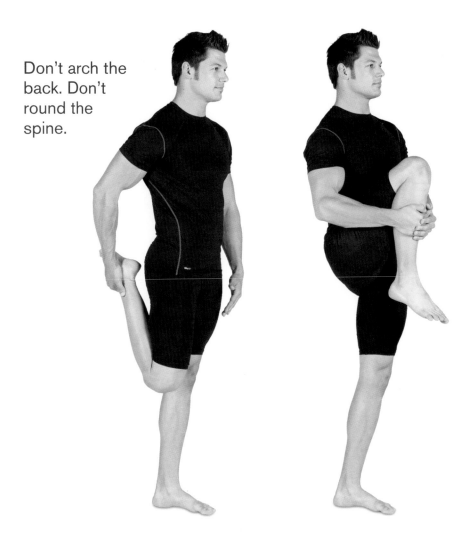

- Stand with the feet shoulder-width apart. Bend one knee and lift the heel toward the gluteals. Hold the ankle with the same-side hand. Release the ankle and move the knee in front of the body as close to the chest as comfortably possible, holding the shin with the hands.

- Return to the start position; repeat the sequence on the other side.

- Each repetition of the sequence should take 2 to 4 seconds and should be performed with controlled momentum. Pause 1 second between repetitions. Repeat the sequence 10 to 12 times.

 breathe **Breathe evenly while performing the sequence.**

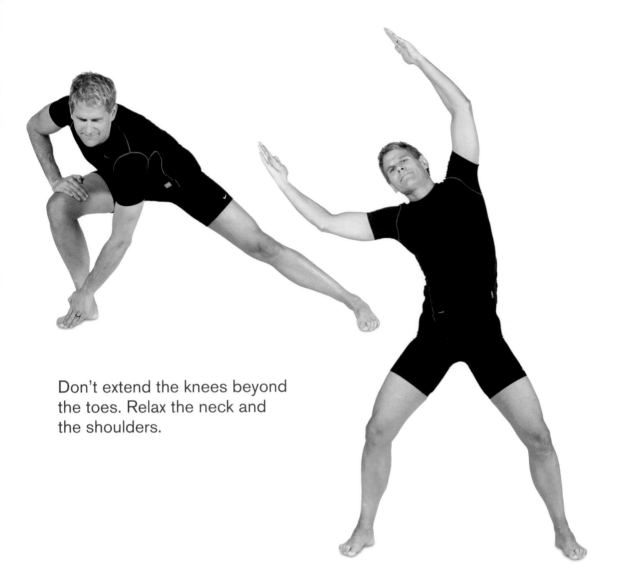

Don't extend the knees beyond the toes. Relax the neck and the shoulders.

- Stand with the feet about 4 feet (1 m) apart. Bend and straighten one knee, lunging to one side. Repeat on the other side.
- Return to the start position. Extending the arms straight overhead, move the arms and the torso in a giant circular motion, clockwise, then counterclockwise.
- Return to the start position.
- Each repetition of the sequence should take 6 to 8 seconds and should be performed with controlled momentum. Pause 1 second between repetitions. Repeat the sequence 10 to 12 times.

breathe **Breathe evenly while performing the sequence.**

part III

Fitness and Sport Routines

General Stretch Routines	
Sport Stretch Routines	
Specialty Stretch Routines	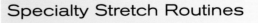

General Stretch Routines

The routines in this chapter are designed to be part of your general fitness program. This chapter includes nine routines in all, ranging from 10 minutes to 40 minutes in duration. Wherever and whenever you choose to work out, one of these routines should fit into your regime and schedule.

For each routine in this section of the book we include a small photo showing each stretch. If you don't recall how to do a particular stretch in a routine, simply turn to the page listed below the photo to refresh your memory.

Express Total-Body Routine

STANDING

This routine is perfect if you want to stretch your whole body but don't have a lot of time. There's nothing fancy here—just simple stretches designed to target the most important muscle groups in a minimum amount of time. Because all the stretches are executed from a standing position, the routine works well outside on damp surfaces as well as in a small or cluttered room where it's inconvenient to move to the floor.

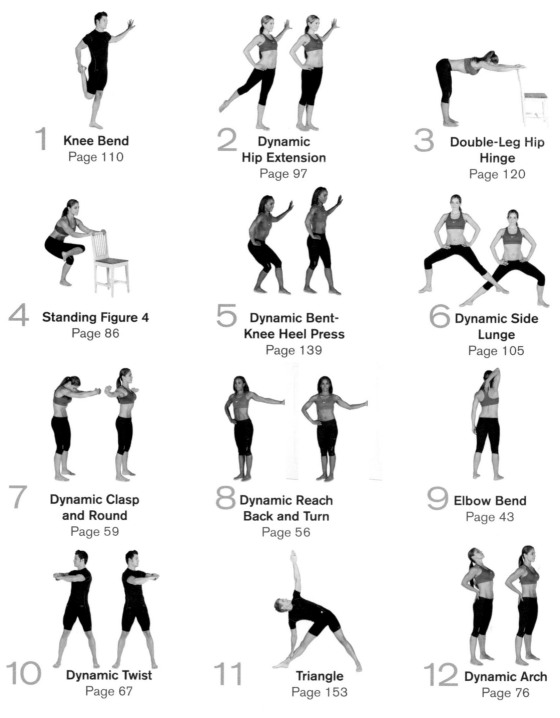

1 **Knee Bend**
Page 110

2 **Dynamic Hip Extension**
Page 97

3 **Double-Leg Hip Hinge**
Page 120

4 **Standing Figure 4**
Page 86

5 **Dynamic Bent-Knee Heel Press**
Page 139

6 **Dynamic Side Lunge**
Page 105

7 **Dynamic Clasp and Round**
Page 59

8 **Dynamic Reach Back and Turn**
Page 56

9 **Elbow Bend**
Page 43

10 **Dynamic Twist**
Page 67

11 **Triangle**
Page 153

12 **Dynamic Arch**
Page 76

SEATED AND LYING

Like the standing express total-body routine, this routine allows you to stretch your entire body when time is limited. Here all stretches are done from a seated or lying position, which is perfect for when you have the space or opportunity to move to the ground or when you have surface areas conducive to stretching on the floor.

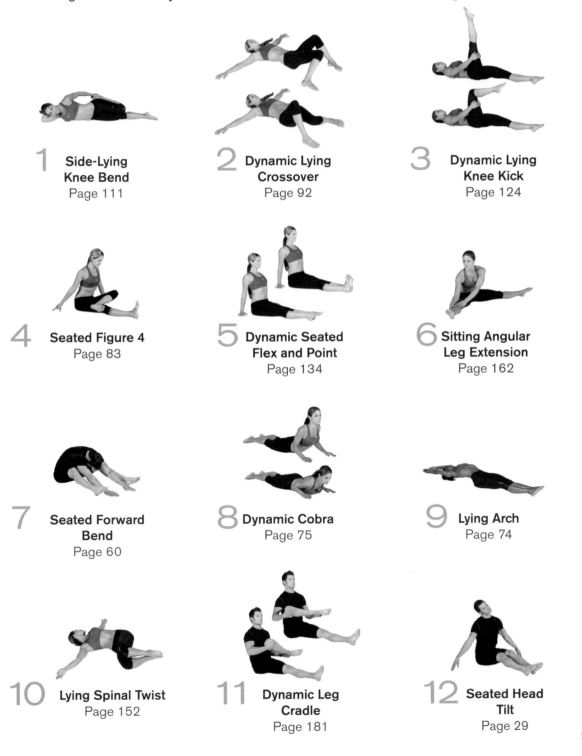

1 **Side-Lying Knee Bend**
Page 111

2 **Dynamic Lying Crossover**
Page 92

3 **Dynamic Lying Knee Kick**
Page 124

4 **Seated Figure 4**
Page 83

5 **Dynamic Seated Flex and Point**
Page 134

6 **Sitting Angular Leg Extension**
Page 162

7 **Seated Forward Bend**
Page 60

8 **Dynamic Cobra**
Page 75

9 **Lying Arch**
Page 74

10 **Lying Spinal Twist**
Page 152

11 **Dynamic Leg Cradle**
Page 181

12 **Seated Head Tilt**
Page 29

Condensed Total-Body Routine

SEATED AND LYING TO STANDING

This routine is for when you have more than 10 minutes but fewer than 40. The sequence here takes you through sitting and lying-down stretches first and then finishes with standing stretches, which makes it a great routine to complete before

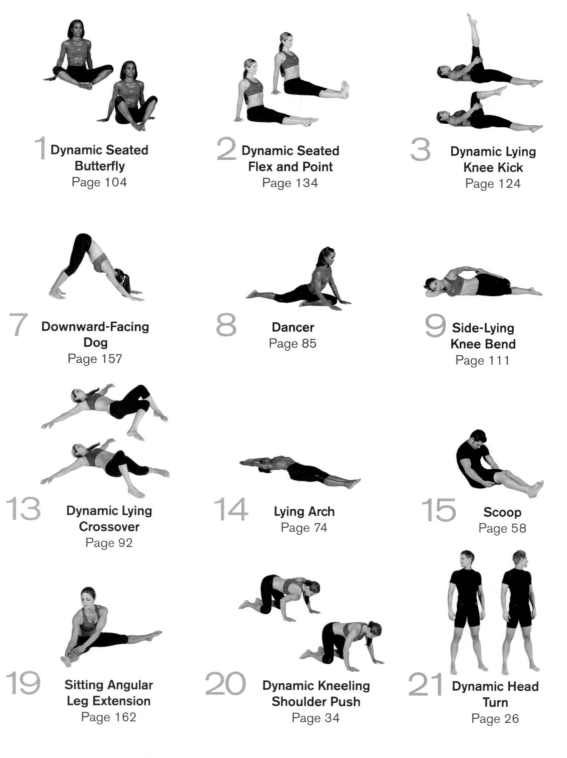

1 **Dynamic Seated Butterfly**
Page 104

2 **Dynamic Seated Flex and Point**
Page 134

3 **Dynamic Lying Knee Kick**
Page 124

7 **Downward-Facing Dog**
Page 157

8 **Dancer**
Page 85

9 **Side-Lying Knee Bend**
Page 111

13 **Dynamic Lying Crossover**
Page 92

14 **Lying Arch**
Page 74

15 **Scoop**
Page 58

19 **Sitting Angular Leg Extension**
Page 162

20 **Dynamic Kneeling Shoulder Push**
Page 34

21 **Dynamic Head Turn**
Page 26

you leave the house or gym. Although this routine doesn't require much time, it contains stretches that are challenging and intense. This is a power-packed routine filled with flowing sequences to balance your body from head to toe.

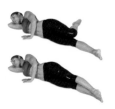 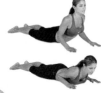

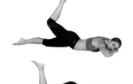 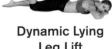

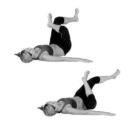

4 **Dynamic Side-Lying Knee Bend**
Page 113

5 **Dynamic Lying Leg Lift**
Page 96

6 **Dynamic Cobra**
Page 75

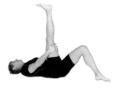 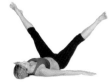 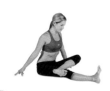

10 **Lying Leg Raise**
Page 118

11 **Lying Straddle**
Page 101

12 **Dynamic Lying Figure-4 Circle**
Page 89

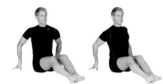 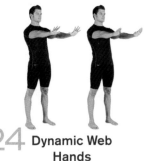

16 **Seated Twist**
Page 66

17 **Dynamic Seated Shoulder Push**
Page 35

18 **Seated Figure 4**
Page 83

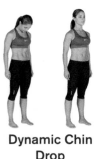 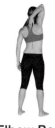

22 **Dynamic Chin Drop**
Page 30

23 **Elbow Bend**
Page 43

24 **Dynamic Web Hands**
Page 49

Condensed Total-Body Routine

STANDING TO SEATED AND LYING

This is another routine for when you have more than 10 minutes but still want to be efficient with your time. Here you begin with stretches from a standing position and finish with stretches that take you to the floor, which makes it an excellent routine to do before settling in for the evening.

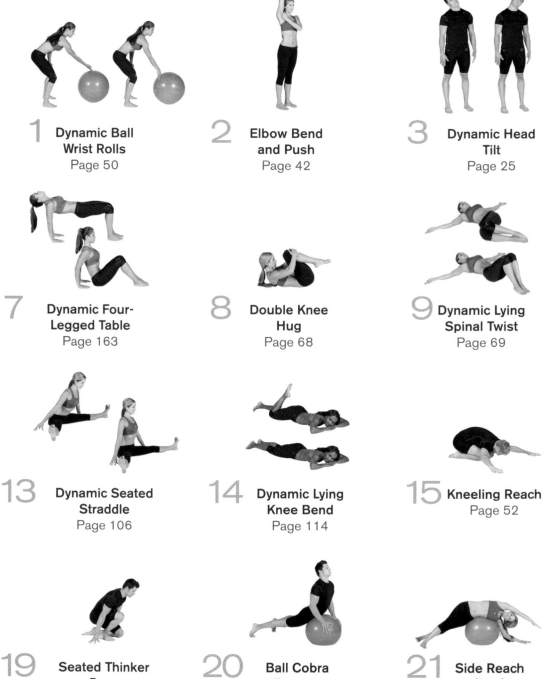

1 **Dynamic Ball Wrist Rolls**
Page 50

2 **Elbow Bend and Push**
Page 42

3 **Dynamic Head Tilt**
Page 25

7 **Dynamic Four-Legged Table**
Page 163

8 **Double Knee Hug**
Page 68

9 **Dynamic Lying Spinal Twist**
Page 69

13 **Dynamic Seated Straddle**
Page 106

14 **Dynamic Lying Knee Bend**
Page 114

15 **Kneeling Reach**
Page 52

19 **Seated Thinker Pose**
Page 136

20 **Ball Cobra**
Page 78

21 **Side Reach (Ball)**
Page 70

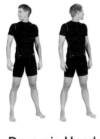

4 Dynamic Head
Turn
Page 26

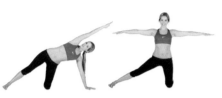

5 Dynamic Half-Circle
Page 182

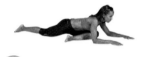

6 Pigeon
Page 183

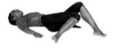

10 Lying Crossover
Page 91

11 Lying Figure 4
Page 82

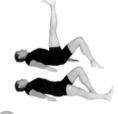

12 Dynamic Lying
Leg Raise
Page 123

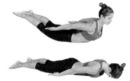

16 Dynamic Grasshopper
Page 170

17 Kneeling Toe
Point and Sit
Page 143

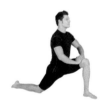

18 Kneeling
Runner's Lunge
Page 94

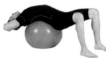

22 Wrap Around Ball
Page 73

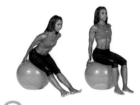

23 Dynamic Rolling
Ball Hip Hinge
Page 127

Complete Total-Body Routine

This is the most challenging and comprehensive routine in the book and should be done when you feel your body needs a complete and thorough stretch release and when you have enough time to devote to a longer routine. You begin this routine standing, work your way to the floor gradually, and move back up to standing at the end of the routine. You'll notice that about 30 minutes into the routine you'll need

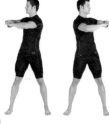

1 **Dynamic Twist**
Page 67

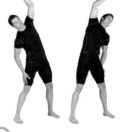

2 **Dynamic Side Reach**
Page 65

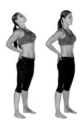

3 **Dynamic Arch**
Page 76

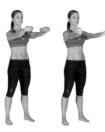

7 **Dynamic Flex and Extend—Wrists**
Page 46

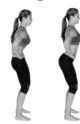

8 **Dynamic Pelvic Tilt**
Page 61

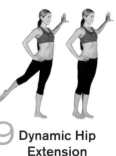

9 **Dynamic Hip Extension**
Page 97

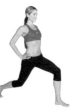

13 **Lunge**
Page 93

14 **Seated Thinker Pose**
Page 136

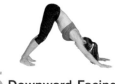

15 **Downward-Facing Dog**
Page 157

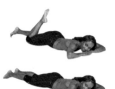

19 **Dynamic Lying Knee Bend**
Page 114

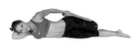

20 **Side-Lying Knee Bend**
Page 111

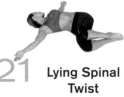

21 **Lying Spinal Twist**
Page 152

a chair to execute some of the stretches. If you want to shorten the routine to 30 minutes, this is a good place to stop. If you're ready to complete the full routine, then grab a chair and continue. You will feel strong, stretched, and centered when you finish this routine.

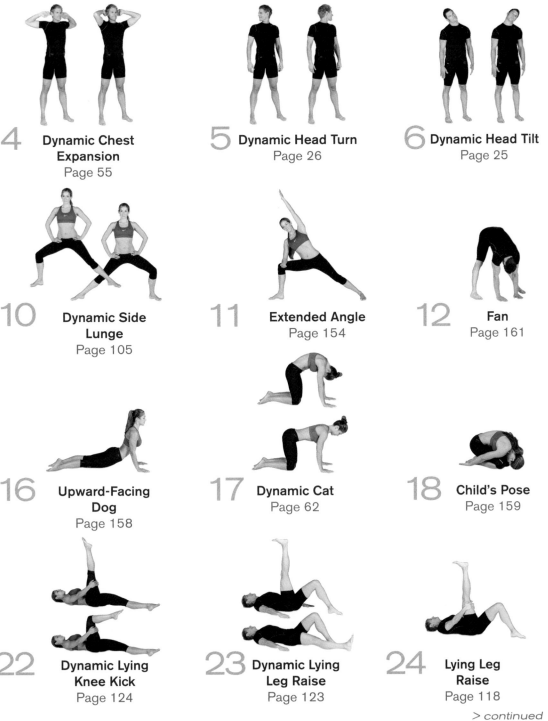

4 **Dynamic Chest Expansion**
Page 55

5 **Dynamic Head Turn**
Page 26

6 **Dynamic Head Tilt**
Page 25

10 **Dynamic Side Lunge**
Page 105

11 **Extended Angle**
Page 154

12 **Fan**
Page 161

16 **Upward-Facing Dog**
Page 158

17 **Dynamic Cat**
Page 62

18 **Child's Pose**
Page 159

22 **Dynamic Lying Knee Kick**
Page 124

23 **Dynamic Lying Leg Raise**
Page 123

24 **Lying Leg Raise**
Page 118

> continued 217

25 Lying Figure 4
Page 82

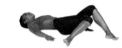

26 Lying Crossover
Page 91

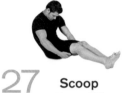

27 Scoop
Page 58

31 Cow Face
Page 172

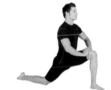

32 Kneeling Runner's
Lunge
Page 94

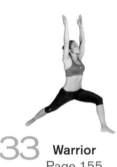

33 Warrior
Page 155

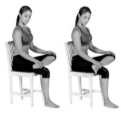

37 Dynamic Seated
Ankle Roll
Page 146

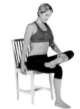

38 Dynamic Seated
Toe Wiggle
Page 149

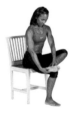

39 Seated Foot
Massage
Page 147

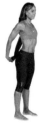

43 Reach Behind
and Open
Page 32

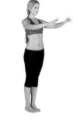

44 Dynamic Piano
Fingers
Page 48

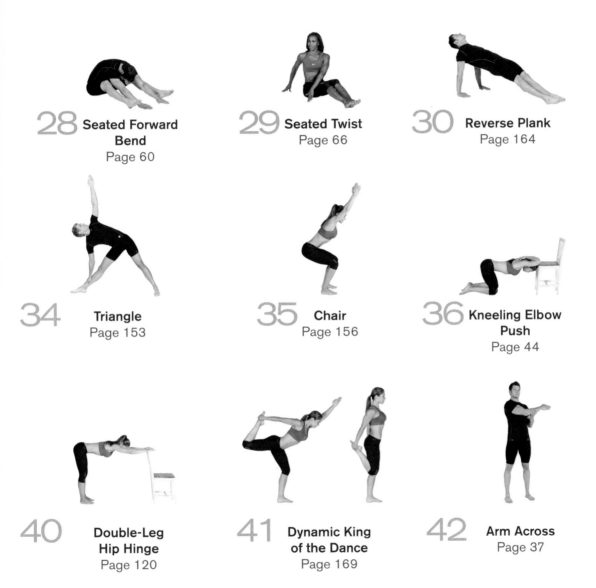

28 Seated Forward
Bend
Page 60

29 Seated Twist
Page 66

30 Reverse Plank
Page 164

34 Triangle
Page 153

35 Chair
Page 156

36 Kneeling Elbow
Push
Page 44

40 Double-Leg
Hip Hinge
Page 120

41 Dynamic King
of the Dance
Page 169

42 Arm Across
Page 37

Strength Training Routine

This routine is designed to complement a traditional total-body strength training program. With stretches to counteract the soreness and tightness that comes from performing exercises such as the bench press, lat pull-down, leg press, biceps curls, hamstring curls, and shoulder press in the weight room, this routine helps you stay flexible while improving your strength.

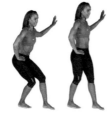

1 Dynamic Bent-Knee
Heel Press
Page 139

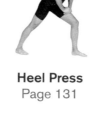

2 Heel Press
Page 131

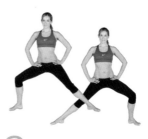

3 Dynamic Side
Lunge
Page 105

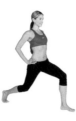

7 Lunge
Page 93

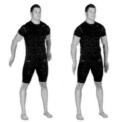

8 Dynamic Rotated
Flyaway
Page 41

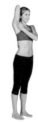

9 Elbow Bend
and Push
Page 42

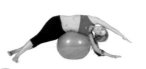

13 Side Reach (Ball)
Page 70

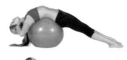

14 Dynamic Supine
Roll Back
Page 77

15 Dynamic Forward
Bend Hip Shift
Page 71

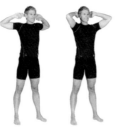

19 Dynamic Chest Expansion
Page 55

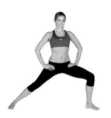

4   **Side Lunge**
Page 99

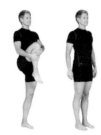

5   **Dynamic Knee Hug**
Page 88

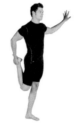

6   **Knee Bend**
Page 110

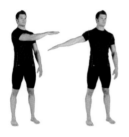

10   **Dynamic Arm Across**
Page 38

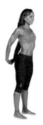

11   **Reach Behind
and Open**
Page 32

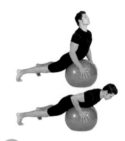

12   **Dynamic Ball
Cobra**
Page 79

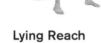
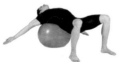

16   **Lying Reach**
Page 57

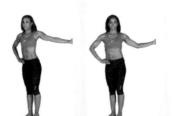

17   **Dynamic Reach
Back and Turn**
Page 56

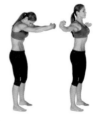

18   **Dynamic Clasp
and Round**
Page 59

Cardiovascular Training Routine

This routine is meant to complement your cardiovascular training program. With stretches designed to counteract the soreness and tightness that comes from working out on a treadmill, elliptical machine, or stair-stepper or from running, swimming, biking, or power walking, this routine helps keep you flexible as you develop your cardiovascular health.

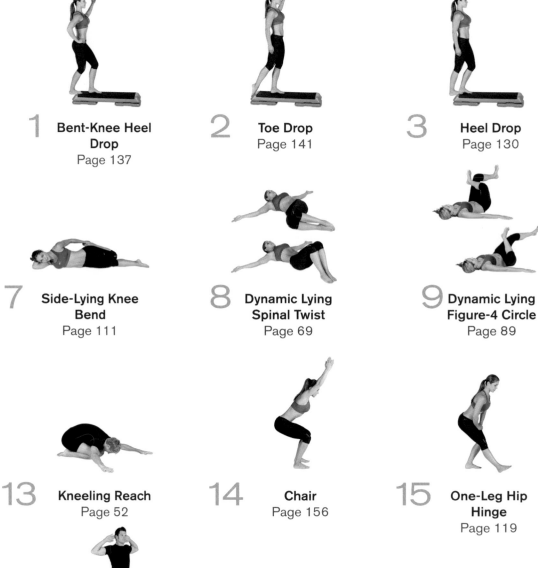

1 Bent-Knee Heel Drop
Page 137

2 Toe Drop
Page 141

3 Heel Drop
Page 130

7 Side-Lying Knee Bend
Page 111

8 Dynamic Lying Spinal Twist
Page 69

9 Dynamic Lying Figure-4 Circle
Page 89

13 Kneeling Reach
Page 52

14 Chair
Page 156

15 One-Leg Hip Hinge
Page 119

19 Chest Expansion
Page 54

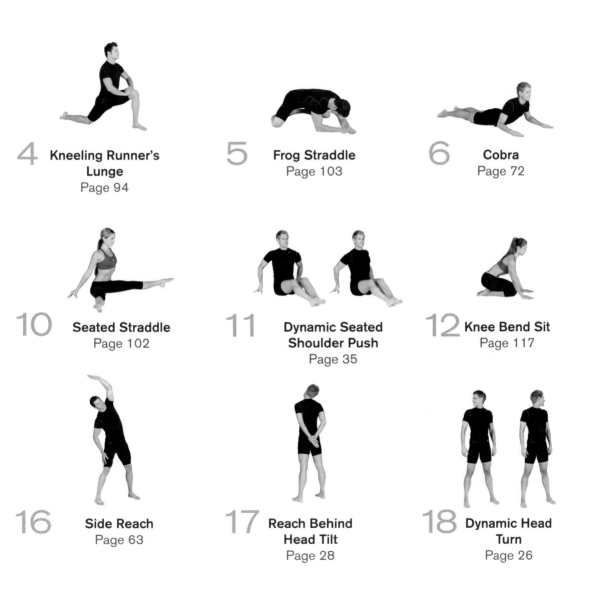

4 **Kneeling Runner's Lunge**
Page 94

5 **Frog Straddle**
Page 103

6 **Cobra**
Page 72

10 **Seated Straddle**
Page 102

11 **Dynamic Seated Shoulder Push**
Page 35

12 **Knee Bend Sit**
Page 117

16 **Side Reach**
Page 63

17 **Reach Behind Head Tilt**
Page 28

18 **Dynamic Head Turn**
Page 26

Made up exclusively of selected stretches inspired by yoga, this routine is short but challenging because most of the stretches focus on multiple muscle groups at the same time and require a degree of strength as well as flexibility. This is an ideal routine for when you are pressed for time but want some of the physical benefits yoga has to offer.

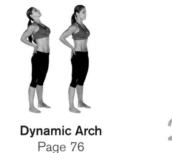

1   **Dynamic Arch**
Page 76

2   **Forward Bend**
Page 160

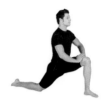

3   **Kneeling Runner's Lunge**
Page 94

7   **Frog**
Page 180

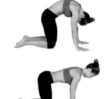

8   **Dynamic Cat**
Page 62

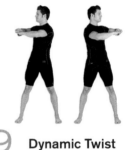

9   **Dynamic Twist**
Page 67

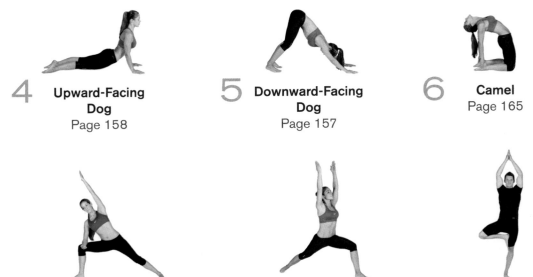

This routine brings together a wide array of stretches inspired by yoga in a flowing sequence that provides a total-body flexibility challenge. The routine requires concentration and effort but makes you feel great and gives you a taste of the benefits of a full-fledged yoga workout.

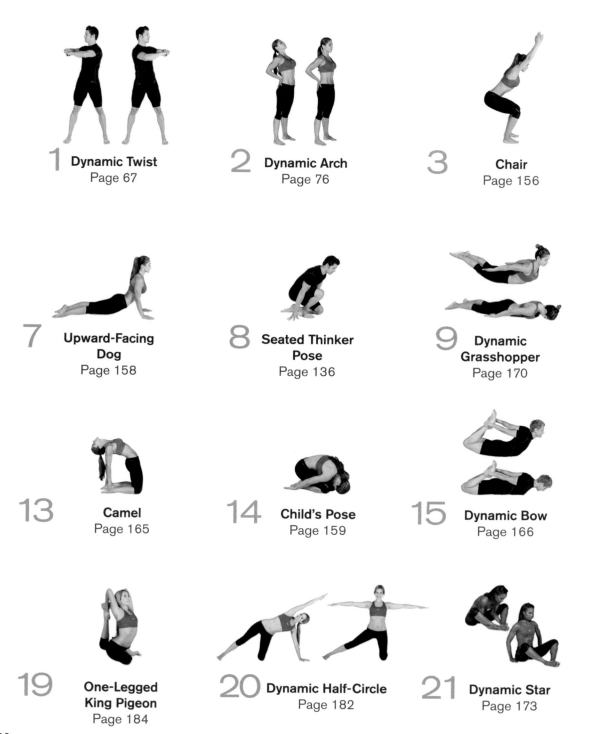

1 Dynamic Twist
Page 67

2 Dynamic Arch
Page 76

3 Chair
Page 156

7 Upward-Facing Dog
Page 158

8 Seated Thinker Pose
Page 136

9 Dynamic Grasshopper
Page 170

13 Camel
Page 165

14 Child's Pose
Page 159

15 Dynamic Bow
Page 166

19 One-Legged King Pigeon
Page 184

20 Dynamic Half-Circle
Page 182

21 Dynamic Star
Page 173

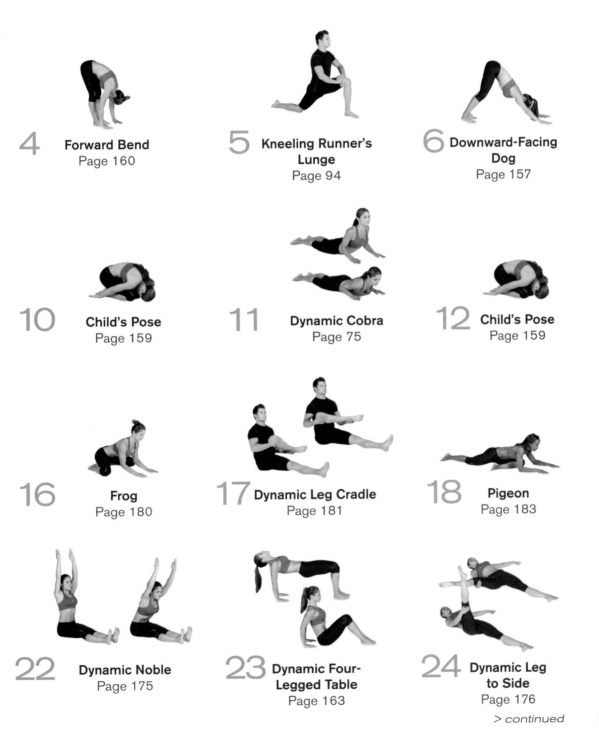

4 Forward Bend
Page 160

5 Kneeling Runner's Lunge
Page 94

6 Downward-Facing Dog
Page 157

10 Child's Pose
Page 159

11 Dynamic Cobra
Page 75

12 Child's Pose
Page 159

16 Frog
Page 180

17 Dynamic Leg Cradle
Page 181

18 Pigeon
Page 183

22 Dynamic Noble
Page 175

23 Dynamic Four-Legged Table
Page 163

24 Dynamic Leg to Side
Page 176

> continued
227

25 **Reverse Plank**
Page 164

26 **Cow Face**
Page 172

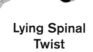

27 **Lying Spinal Twist**
Page 152

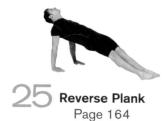

31 **Downward-Facing Dog**
Page 157

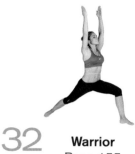

32 **Warrior**
Page 155

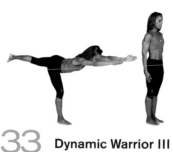

33 **Dynamic Warrior III**
Page 167

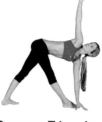

37 **Reverse Triangle**
Page 171

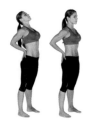

38 **Dynamic Arch**
Page 76

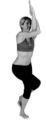

39 **Eagle**
Page 168

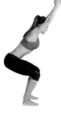

43 **Chair**
Page 156

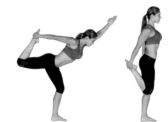

44 **Dynamic King of the Dance**
Page 169

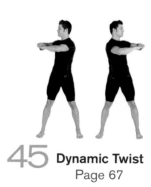

45 **Dynamic Twist**
Page 67

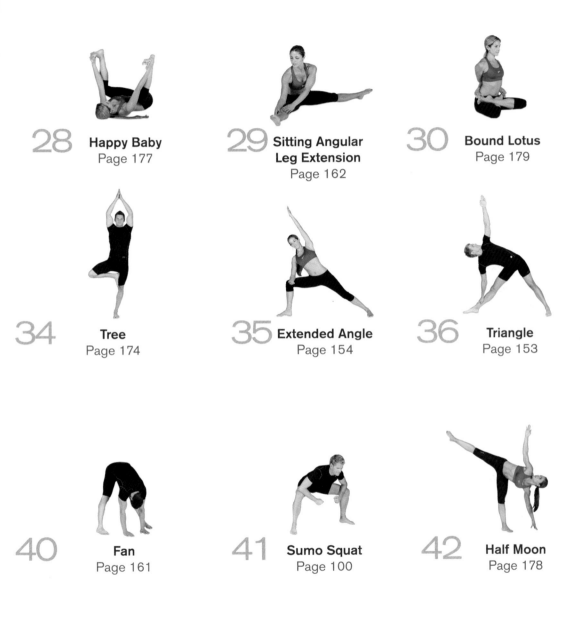

28 **Happy Baby**
Page 177

29 **Sitting Angular
Leg Extension**
Page 162

30 **Bound Lotus**
Page 179

34 **Tree**
Page 174

35 **Extended Angle**
Page 154

36 **Triangle**
Page 153

40 **Fan**
Page 161

41 **Sumo Squat**
Page 100

42 **Half Moon**
Page 178

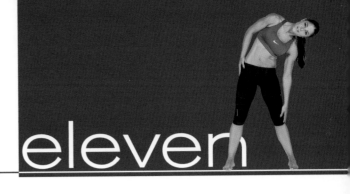

eleven

Sport Stretch Routines

This chapter presents stretch routines for a series of sport applications, including routines for warming up and cooling down, routines for three major categories of sport, and routines made up exclusively of sport mobility stretches from chapter 9.

Each routine is designed to improve the range of motion in joints that are active when playing a variety of sports and to release tension in muscles that tend to be overworked or fatigued through sport participation.

Warm-Up Stretch Routine

This routine focuses primarily on dynamic stretches that warm up your body and prepare you for a variety of sports. These stretches are not sport-specific, but performing them before practice or a game will enhance total-body range of motion, increase tissue temperature, and reduce the injury risk.

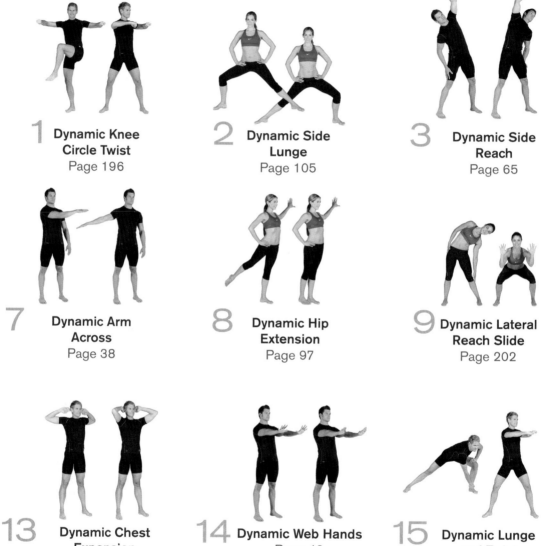

1 Dynamic Knee
Circle Twist
Page 196

2 Dynamic Side
Lunge
Page 105

3 Dynamic Side
Reach
Page 65

7 Dynamic Arm
Across
Page 38

8 Dynamic Hip
Extension
Page 97

9 Dynamic Lateral
Reach Slide
Page 202

13 Dynamic Chest
Expansion
Page 55

14 Dynamic Web Hands
Page 49

15 Dynamic Lunge
and Twist
Page 194

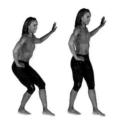

4 Dynamic Bent-Knee
Heel Press
Page 139

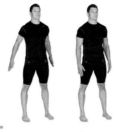

5 Dynamic Flyaway
Page 33

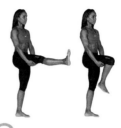

6 Dynamic Knee
Kick
Page 122

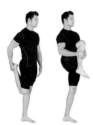

10 Dynamic Knee Bend
and Hug
Page 204

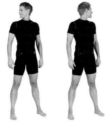

11 Dynamic Head Turn
Page 26

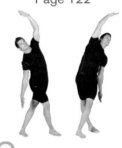

12 Dynamic Cross-
Reach
Page 191

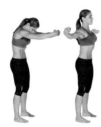

16 Dynamic Clasp
and Round
Page 59

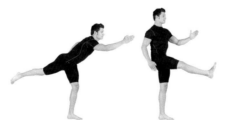

17 Dynamic Straight-Leg
Pendulum
Page 186

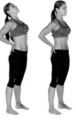

18 Dynamic Arch
Page 76

This routine emphasizes static-passive stretches that lengthen and relax sore and tired muscles following a tough practice or athletic contest. These stretches won't necessarily improve sport performance, but they will increase your range of motion and help you achieve and maintain the flexibility required to be a good athlete while keeping your body tuned up and injury free.

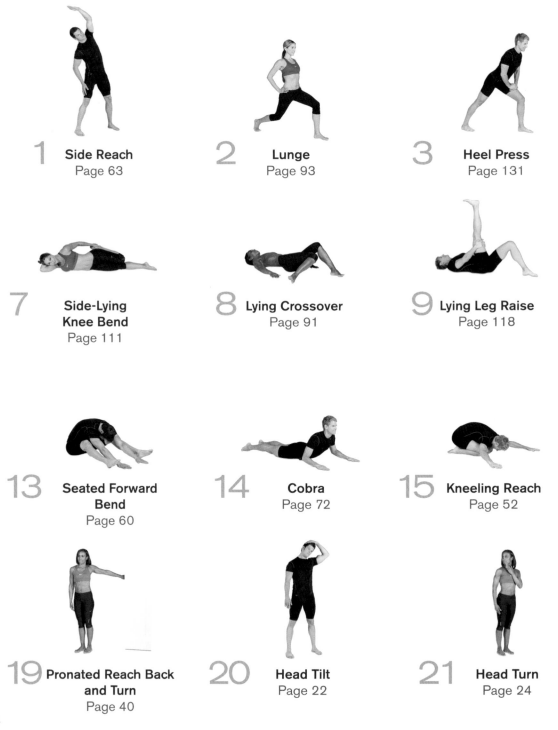

1 **Side Reach**
Page 63

2 **Lunge**
Page 93

3 **Heel Press**
Page 131

7 **Side-Lying Knee Bend**
Page 111

8 **Lying Crossover**
Page 91

9 **Lying Leg Raise**
Page 118

13 **Seated Forward Bend**
Page 60

14 **Cobra**
Page 72

15 **Kneeling Reach**
Page 52

19 **Pronated Reach Back and Turn**
Page 40

20 **Head Tilt**
Page 22

21 **Head Turn**
Page 24

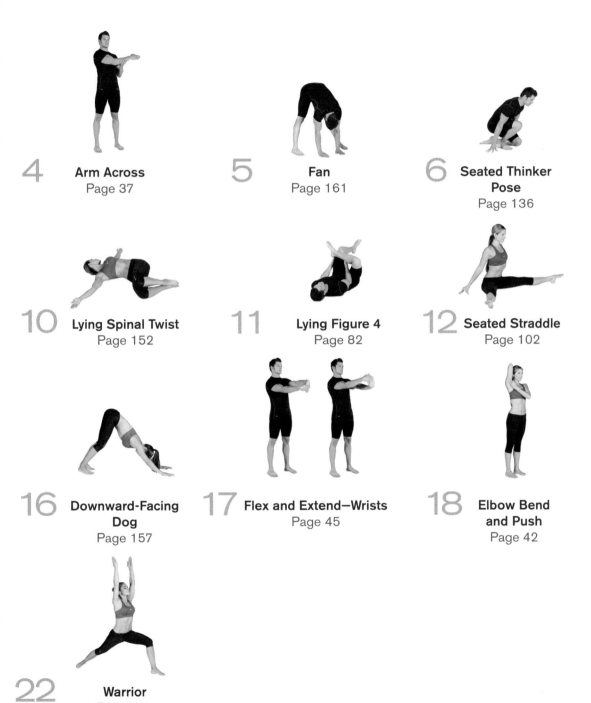

4 **Arm Across**
Page 37

5 **Fan**
Page 161

6 **Seated Thinker
Pose**
Page 136

10 **Lying Spinal Twist**
Page 152

11 **Lying Figure 4**
Page 82

12 **Seated Straddle**
Page 102

16 **Downward-Facing
Dog**
Page 157

17 **Flex and Extend—Wrists**
Page 45

18 **Elbow Bend
and Push**
Page 42

22 **Warrior**
Page 155

This routine uses exclusively the sport mobility stretches presented in chapter 9. Because the stretches are designed to simulate common sport movement patterns, this routine is ideal for keeping you sport-ready during the off-season.

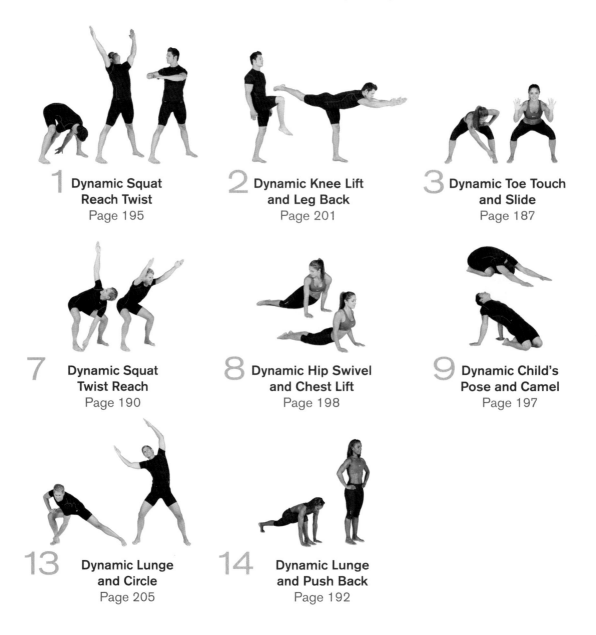

1 Dynamic Squat
Reach Twist
Page 195

2 Dynamic Knee Lift
and Leg Back
Page 201

3 Dynamic Toe Touch
and Slide
Page 187

7 Dynamic Squat
Twist Reach
Page 190

8 Dynamic Hip Swivel
and Chest Lift
Page 198

9 Dynamic Child's
Pose and Camel
Page 197

13 Dynamic Lunge
and Circle
Page 205

14 Dynamic Lunge
and Push Back
Page 192

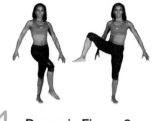

4 **Dynamic Figure 8**
Page 203

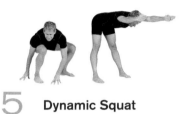

5 **Dynamic Squat
Twist and Hinge**
Page 200

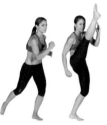

6 **Dynamic Leg Kick**
Page 188

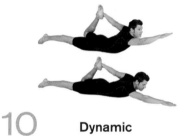

10 **Dynamic
Single-Side Bow**
Page 193

11 **Dynamic Roll
and Reach**
Page 199

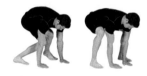

12 **Dynamic Cross-
Knee Squat**
Page 189

This routine combines most of the sport mobility stretches in chapter 9 and is designed to provide a total-body athletic challenge to make you sweat and keep your body loose, reactive, and sport-ready during peak season.

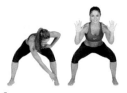

1 **Dynamic Toe Touch and Slide**
Page 187

2 **Dynamic Knee Bend and Hug**
Page 204

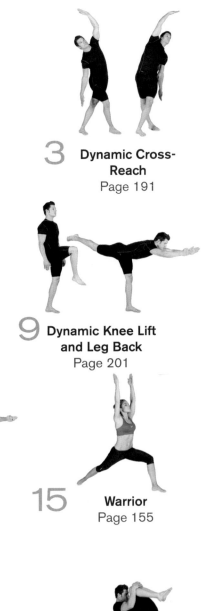

3 **Dynamic Cross-Reach**
Page 191

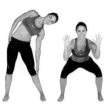

7 **Dynamic Lateral Reach Slide**
Page 202

8 **Dynamic Cross-Knee Squat**
Page 189

9 **Dynamic Knee Lift and Leg Back**
Page 201

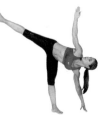

13 **Half Moon**
Page 178

14 **Dynamic Squat Twist and Hinge**
Page 200

15 **Warrior**
Page 155

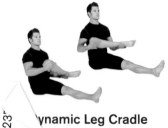

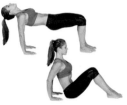

ynamic Leg Cradle
Page 181

20 **Dynamic Four-Legged Table**
Page 163

21 **Dynamic Roll and Reach**
Page 199

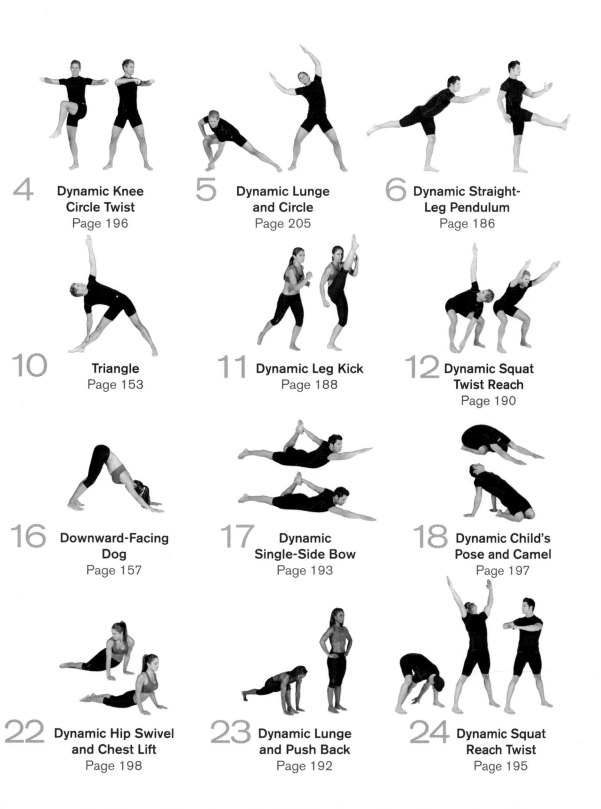

4 **Dynamic Knee Circle Twist**
Page 196

5 **Dynamic Lunge and Circle**
Page 205

6 **Dynamic Straight-Leg Pendulum**
Page 186

10 **Triangle**
Page 153

11 **Dynamic Leg Kick**
Page 188

12 **Dynamic Squat Twist Reach**
Page 190

16 **Downward-Facing Dog**
Page 157

17 **Dynamic Single-Side Bow**
Page 193

18 **Dynamic Child's Pose and Camel**
Page 197

22 **Dynamic Hip Swivel and Chest Lift**
Page 198

23 **Dynamic Lunge and Push Back**
Page 192

24 **Dynamic Squat Reach Twist**
Page 195

Swinging and Throwing Sports Routine

Tennis, squash, racquetball, badminton, table tennis, golf, baseball, softball, cricket, curling, water polo, bowling

Swinging and throwing sports typically emphasize the upper body. This doesn't mean the lower body is not important in these activities but that flexibility and strength of the upper body is most critical. In swinging and throwing sports, the muscles of

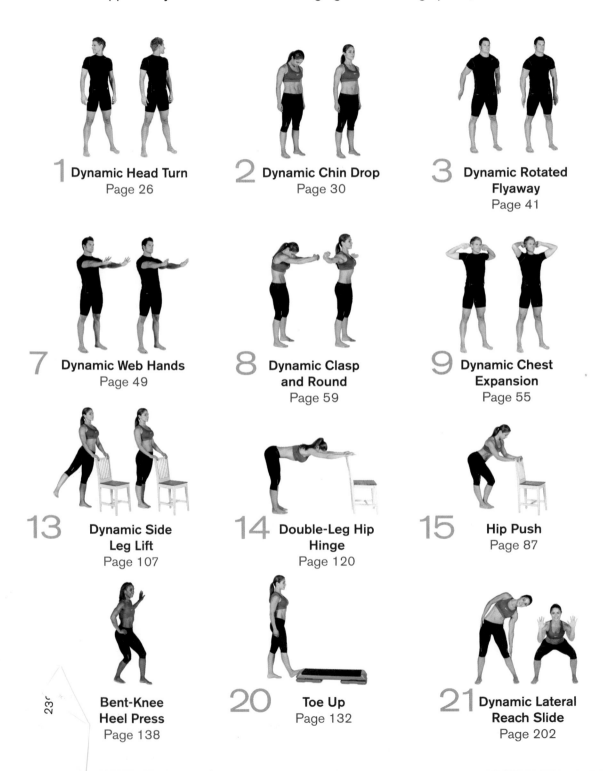

1 **Dynamic Head Turn**
Page 26

2 **Dynamic Chin Drop**
Page 30

3 **Dynamic Rotated Flyaway**
Page 41

7 **Dynamic Web Hands**
Page 49

8 **Dynamic Clasp and Round**
Page 59

9 **Dynamic Chest Expansion**
Page 55

13 **Dynamic Side Leg Lift**
Page 107

14 **Double-Leg Hip Hinge**
Page 120

15 **Hip Push**
Page 87

Bent-Knee Heel Press
Page 138

20 **Toe Up**
Page 132

21 **Dynamic Lateral Reach Slide**
Page 202

the neck, shoulders, arms, and torso are constantly challenged and require a great deal of mobility. This stretch routine is the perfect complement for these activities.

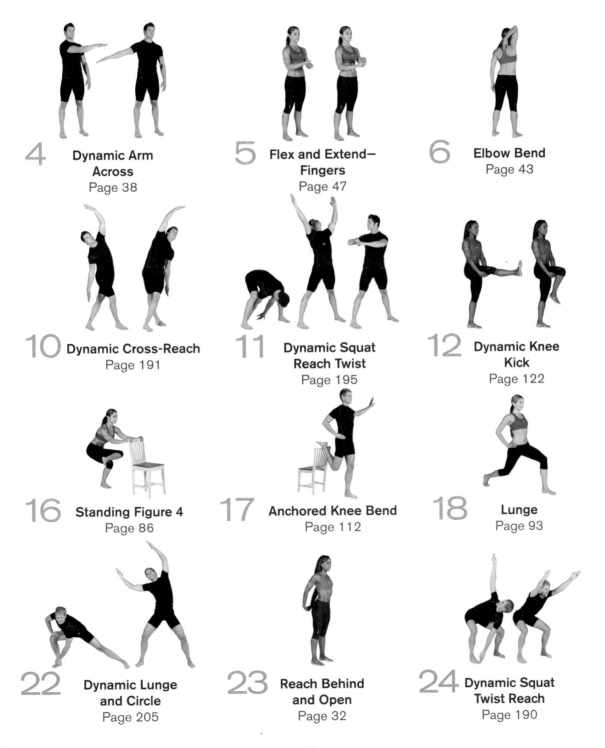

4 **Dynamic Arm Across**
Page 38

5 **Flex and Extend— Fingers**
Page 47

6 **Elbow Bend**
Page 43

10 **Dynamic Cross-Reach**
Page 191

11 **Dynamic Squat Reach Twist**
Page 195

12 **Dynamic Knee Kick**
Page 122

16 **Standing Figure 4**
Page 86

17 **Anchored Knee Bend**
Page 112

18 **Lunge**
Page 93

22 **Dynamic Lunge and Circle**
Page 205

23 **Reach Behind and Open**
Page 32

24 **Dynamic Squat Twist Reach**
Page 190

Endurance and Distance Sports Routine

Running, walking, cross-country skiing, cycling, field hockey, rowing, soccer, kayaking, lacrosse, rock climbing, Australian rules football, swimming

In endurance and distance sports, a key factor is sustaining the activity over time, usually with an emphasis on the lower-body muscles. Grouping soccer and rock climbing into the same category might seem strange, but both activities require

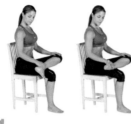

1 Dynamic Seated Half-Circle
Page 144

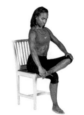

2 Seated Foot Pull
Page 142

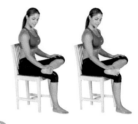

3 Dynamic Seated Toe Flex and Point
Page 148

7 Seated Stretch-Strap Foot Pull
Page 133

8 Dynamic Roll and Reach
Page 199

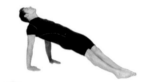

9 Reverse Plank
Page 164

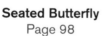

13 Seated Butterfly
Page 98

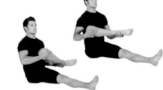

14 Dynamic Leg Cradle
Page 181

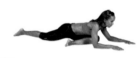

15 Pigeon
Page 183

19 Dynamic Cross-Knee Squat
Page 189

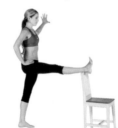

20 Standing Leg Raise
Page 121

21 Dynamic Heel Drop
Page 135

sustained muscular activity over time as well as great power and strength from the lower body. This routine makes all endurance and distance sports easier to complete and also reduces recovery time between events or contests.

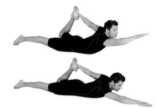

4 **Dynamic Seated
Ankle Pull**
Page 145

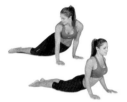

5 **Dynamic Hip Swivel
and Chest Lift**
Page 198

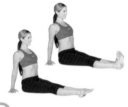

6 **Dynamic Seated
Flex and Point**
Page 134

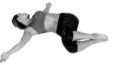

10 **Lying Spinal Twist**
Page 152

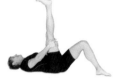

11 **Lying Leg Raise**
Page 118

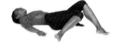

12 **Lying Crossover**
Page 91

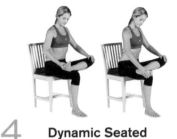

16 **Dynamic
Single-Side Bow**
Page 193

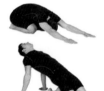

17 **Dynamic Child's
Pose and Camel**
Page 197

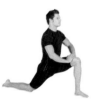

18 **Kneeling
Runner's Lunge**
Page 94

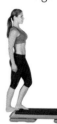

22 **Heel Drop**
Page 130

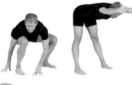

23 **Dynamic Squat
Twist and Hinge**
Page 200

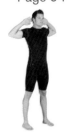

24 **Chest Expansion**
Page 54

Power and Jumping Sports Routine

Boxing, wrestling, martial arts, basketball, volleyball, American football, rugby, ice hockey, netball, gymnastics, figure skating, surfing, snowboarding, snow skiing, water skiing

All power and jumping sports require explosive force and strength. Whether you're kicking in karate, tumbling in gymnastics, or jumping in basketball, the muscles must fire quickly and powerfully, usually in short bursts rather than sustained efforts. The

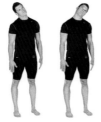

1 **Dynamic Head Tilt**
Page 25

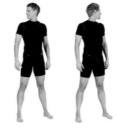

2 **Dynamic Head Turn**
Page 26

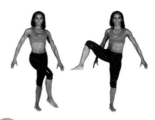

3 **Dynamic Figure 8**
Page 203

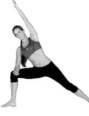

7 **Extended Angle**
Page 154

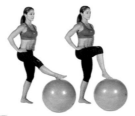

8 **Dynamic Rolling
Ball Knee Kick**
Page 126

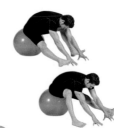

9 **Dynamic Forward
Bend Hip Shift**
Page 71

13 **Lying Crossover**
Page 91

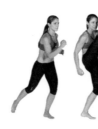

14 **Dynamic Lying
Leg Raise**
Page 123

15 **Dynamic Lying
Figure-4 Circle**
Page 89

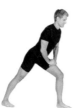

19 **Heel Press**
Page 131

20 **Dynamic Leg Kick**
Page 188

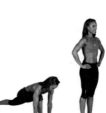

21 **Dynamic Lunge
and Push Back**
Page 192

power and jumping sequence helps build the mobility you need to excel in these sports while reducing the risk of injury along the way.

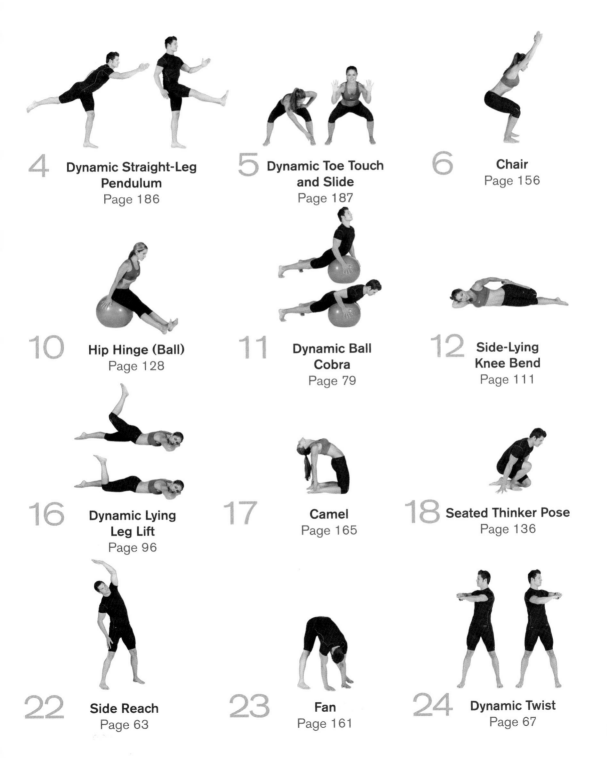

4 **Dynamic Straight-Leg Pendulum**
Page 186

5 **Dynamic Toe Touch and Slide**
Page 187

6 **Chair**
Page 156

10 **Hip Hinge (Ball)**
Page 128

11 **Dynamic Ball Cobra**
Page 79

12 **Side-Lying Knee Bend**
Page 111

16 **Dynamic Lying Leg Lift**
Page 96

17 **Camel**
Page 165

18 **Seated Thinker Pose**
Page 136

22 **Side Reach**
Page 63

23 **Fan**
Page 161

24 **Dynamic Twist**
Page 67

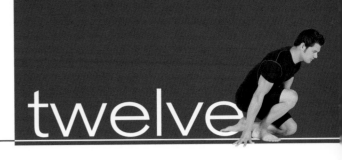
Specialty Stretch Routines

In this chapter each routine has a particular purpose. One is designed to help with lower back problems, another to loosen tight shoulders and neck muscles. There's a routine for the upper body, one for the lower body, and one to help with everyday bending, reaching, and playing. One routine is designed to be used at work and another to improve posture. I love these routines because they fit so conveniently into life. It's easy to make time for a few minutes' worth of stretching. And the payoffs are immediate and real. These routines make you feel energized, relaxed, and prepared for the day to come. They are my favorite routines, and I bet they'll be yours too.

Healthy Back Routine

This routine strengthens and stretches the most important muscles in your trunk and core. You'll have a healthier back and improved posture. If you have chronic back pain, be sure to consult your physician before attempting this routine because some of the stretches are challenging. You'll begin standing, then do some stretches from a chair, and finally work from a seated position on the floor. This is a valuable sequence to do anytime during the day or in conjunction with other routines.

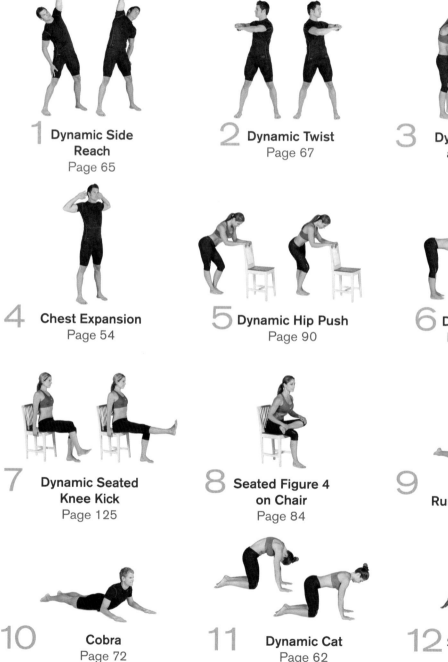

1 **Dynamic Side Reach**
Page 65

2 **Dynamic Twist**
Page 67

3 **Dynamic Clasp and Round**
Page 59

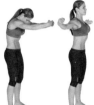

4 **Chest Expansion**
Page 54

5 **Dynamic Hip Push**
Page 90

6 **Double-Leg Hip Hinge**
Page 120

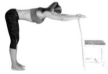

7 **Dynamic Seated Knee Kick**
Page 125

8 **Seated Figure 4 on Chair**
Page 84

9 **Kneeling Runner's Lunge**
Page 94

10 **Cobra**
Page 72

11 **Dynamic Cat**
Page 62

12 **Seated Twist**
Page 66

This routine is ideal if you experience a tight neck or carry your stress in your shoulder area. It's a simple routine that takes only five minutes and that can be done at your desk during the day. When you do this routine, you'll notice your shoulders and neck immediately feel more relaxed, which usually makes it easier to concentrate. Do this routine as often as you like whenever you need a quick break or feel yourself slouching at your desk.

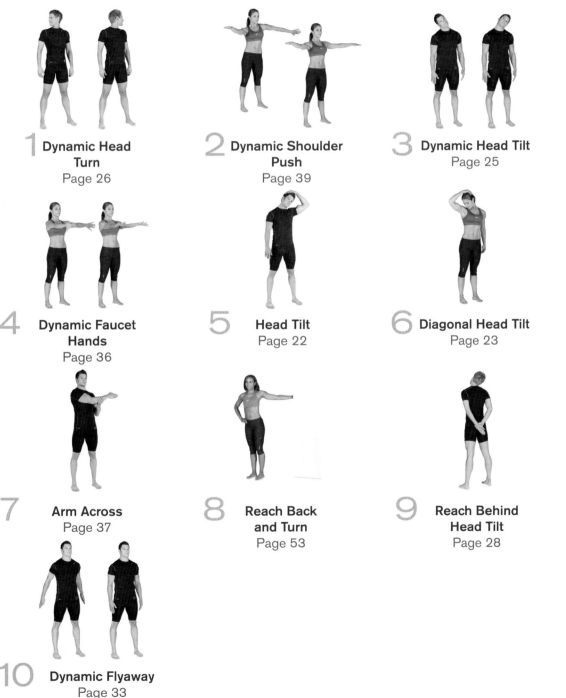

1 **Dynamic Head Turn**
Page 26

2 **Dynamic Shoulder Push**
Page 39

3 **Dynamic Head Tilt**
Page 25

4 **Dynamic Faucet Hands**
Page 36

5 **Head Tilt**
Page 22

6 **Diagonal Head Tilt**
Page 23

7 **Arm Across**
Page 37

8 **Reach Back and Turn**
Page 53

9 **Reach Behind Head Tilt**
Page 28

10 **Dynamic Flyaway**
Page 33

This routine focuses on the muscles above the waist and hip. Try this routine if you use your upper body frequently during the day or if you have done an activity that stresses the upper body, such as snow shoveling, painting, or washing your car.

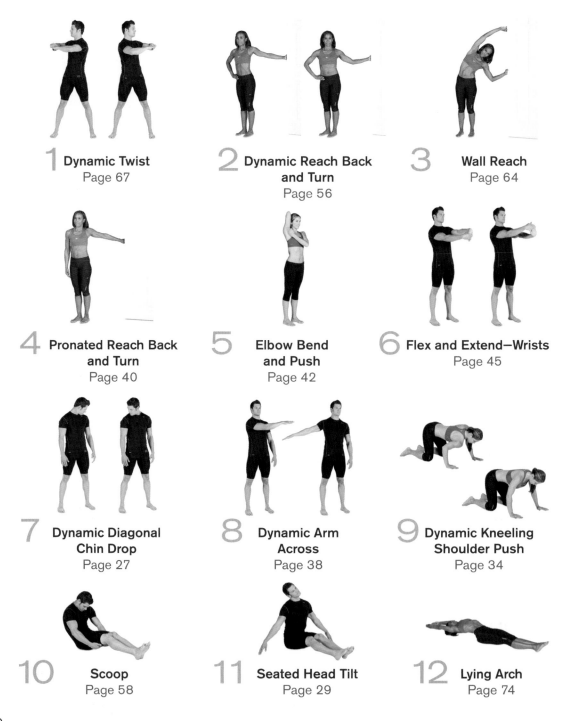

1 **Dynamic Twist**
Page 67

2 **Dynamic Reach Back and Turn**
Page 56

3 **Wall Reach**
Page 64

4 **Pronated Reach Back and Turn**
Page 40

5 **Elbow Bend and Push**
Page 42

6 **Flex and Extend—Wrists**
Page 45

7 **Dynamic Diagonal Chin Drop**
Page 27

8 **Dynamic Arm Across**
Page 38

9 **Dynamic Kneeling Shoulder Push**
Page 34

10 **Scoop**
Page 58

11 **Seated Head Tilt**
Page 29

12 **Lying Arch**
Page 74

This routine is for the muscles below the waist and hips. Try this one if you use your lower body during the day or have done an activity that stresses the lower body, such as climbing stairs, playing chase, or hiking.

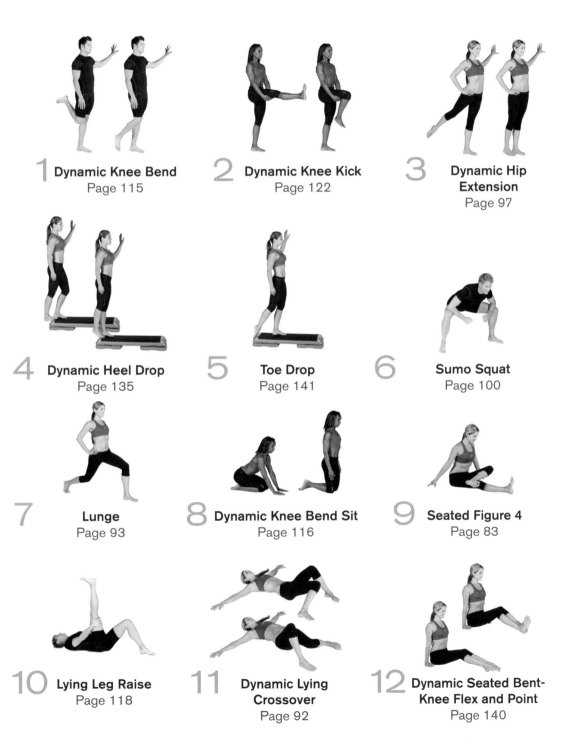

1 **Dynamic Knee Bend**
Page 115

2 **Dynamic Knee Kick**
Page 122

3 **Dynamic Hip Extension**
Page 97

4 **Dynamic Heel Drop**
Page 135

5 **Toe Drop**
Page 141

6 **Sumo Squat**
Page 100

7 **Lunge**
Page 93

8 **Dynamic Knee Bend Sit**
Page 116

9 **Seated Figure 4**
Page 83

10 **Lying Leg Raise**
Page 118

11 **Dynamic Lying Crossover**
Page 92

12 **Dynamic Seated Bent-Knee Flex and Point**
Page 140

This routine makes it easier for you to bend, reach, and play. If you want to improve your ability to get around, play with your kids, or just do simple everyday tasks such as gardening or washing the car, this is a good routine for you. You can do the sequence just once or, ideally, repeat it three to five times in a row, which of course takes much longer but is well worth it. You might be surprised how such a simple routine makes you feel so much better.

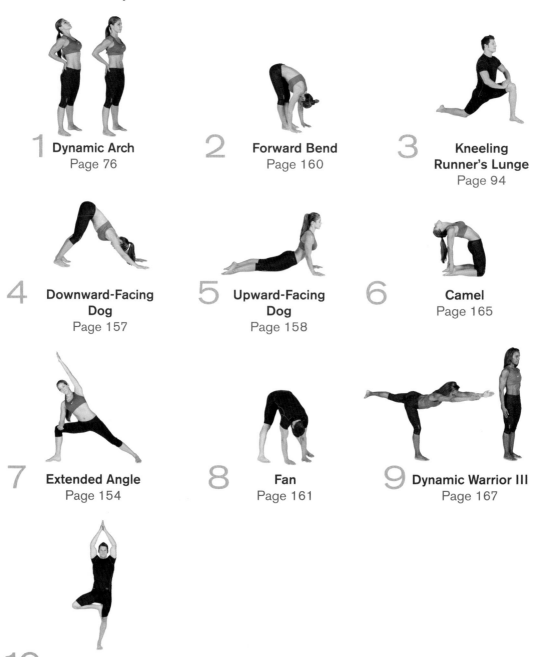

1 **Dynamic Arch**
Page 76

2 **Forward Bend**
Page 160

3 **Kneeling Runner's Lunge**
Page 94

4 **Downward-Facing Dog**
Page 157

5 **Upward-Facing Dog**
Page 158

6 **Camel**
Page 165

7 **Extended Angle**
Page 154

8 **Fan**
Page 161

9 **Dynamic Warrior III**
Page 167

10 **Tree**
Page 174

At-the-Office Routine

This routine can be done easily and quickly at the office at your desk. All the stretches can be done from a standing or seated position. The routine is short but helps reduce back pain and energize your spine.

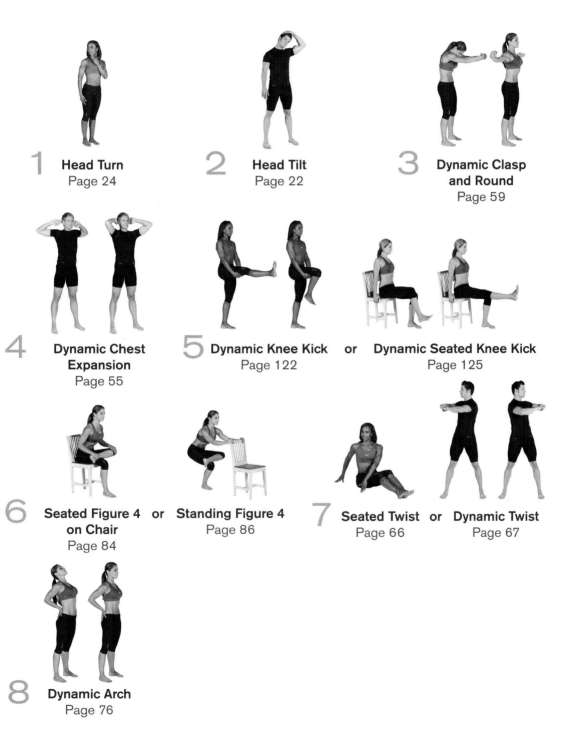

1 **Head Turn**
Page 24

2 **Head Tilt**
Page 22

3 **Dynamic Clasp and Round**
Page 59

4 **Dynamic Chest Expansion**
Page 55

5 **Dynamic Knee Kick** or **Dynamic Seated Knee Kick**
Page 122 / Page 125

6 **Seated Figure 4 on Chair** or **Standing Figure 4**
Page 84 / Page 86

7 **Seated Twist** or **Dynamic Twist**
Page 66 / Page 67

8 **Dynamic Arch**
Page 76

Improved-Posture Routine

Lower back pain is one of the most common ailments and can be exacerbated or caused by poor posture. Many activities, including driving and sitting at a desk, contribute to poor posture. The stretches in this routine will improve posture and strengthen the back.

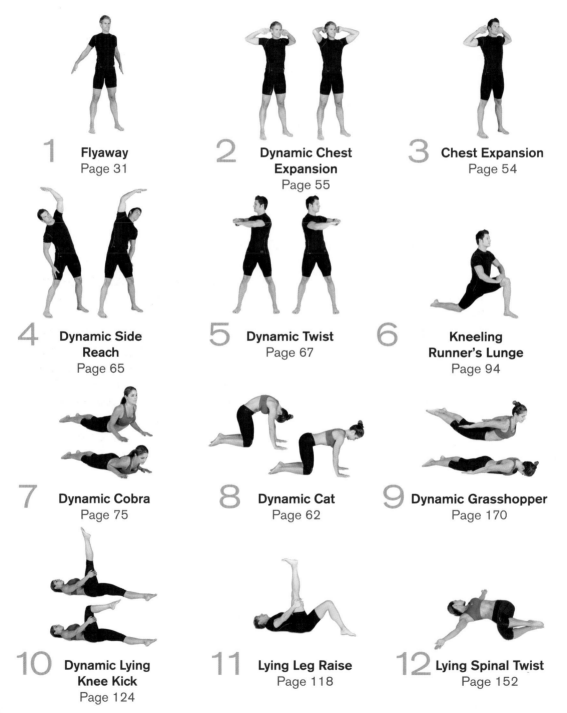

1 **Flyaway**
Page 31

2 **Dynamic Chest Expansion**
Page 55

3 **Chest Expansion**
Page 54

4 **Dynamic Side Reach**
Page 65

5 **Dynamic Twist**
Page 67

6 **Kneeling Runner's Lunge**
Page 94

7 **Dynamic Cobra**
Page 75

8 **Dynamic Cat**
Page 62

9 **Dynamic Grasshopper**
Page 170

10 **Dynamic Lying Knee Kick**
Page 124

11 **Lying Leg Raise**
Page 118

12 **Lying Spinal Twist**
Page 152

about the author

Jay Blahnik is recognized as one of the premier fitness professionals in the industry and has over 25 years of teaching and training experience. As a fitness educator and keynote speaker, he has traveled to over 30 countries and is known for his insightful viewpoints on engaging and motivating consumers.

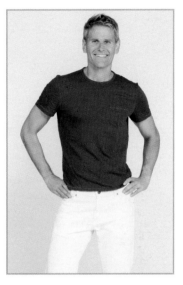

Jay was chosen by *Shape* magazine as one of the top fitness instructors in the world, and *Men's Health* listed him as having one of the top 10 workouts of all time. He is the youngest person ever to receive both the IDEA Fitness Instructor of the Year Award and IDEA's Fitness Industry Icons and Innovators title. He was also chosen as Can-Fit-Pro's International Presenter of the Year in 2005.

He has starred in over 30 award-winning exercise videos and has designed, created, and choreographed some of the best-selling exercise videos of all time for other fitness professionals and celebrities.

Jay has been featured as a fitness expert in over 200 magazines across the globe, and his weekly and monthly fitness columns in the *Los Angeles Times* and on MSNBC.com are read by millions of people each year. He has served as an editorial advisory board member for the American Council on Exercise (ACE) and is the group exercise spokesperson for IDEA Health and Fitness Association.

Jay is a consultant and program developer for Nike, Nautilus, Bowflex, Schwinn, Stairmaster, BOSU, and Indo-Row. He resides in Laguna Beach, California.

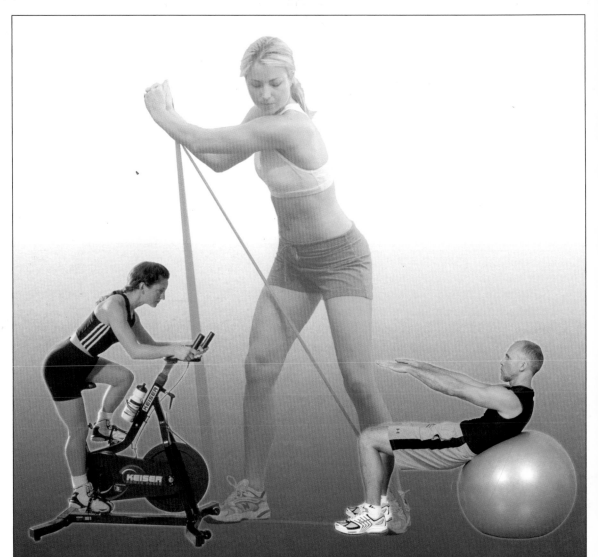

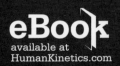